YOGA FOR ALL FOUR PARADIGMS

BHAKTI | KARAM | DHYAN | GYAN

VINOD MALHOTRA

EBD

EMBASSY BOOKS
www.embassybooks.in

First Edition 2025,
Published in India by:
Embassy Book Distributors
120, Great Western Building, Maharashtra Chamber of Commerce
Lane, Fort, Mumbai 400 023, India
Tel: (+9122) -30967415, 22819546
Email: info@embassybooks.in
www.embassybooks.in

ISBN: 978-81-19727-21-6

Distribution Centres:
Mumbai, Ahmedabad, Bangalore, Kolkata, Chennai,
Hyderabad, New Delhi, Pune

Cover Design by Rishikumar Thakur for Embassy Book Distributors

Printed & bound in India by Repro India Ltd., Navi Mumbai

YOGA FOR ALL FOUR PARADIGMS

BHAKTI | KARAM | DHYAN | GYAN

Table of Contents

PREFACE

Science of Yoga is One of the greatest gifts to mankind by Hinduism, Vedanta civilisation and its age-old Indian traditions. Some modern-day theistic religions such as Judaism, Christianity, Islam, Baha'i Faith, Sikhism, Zoroastrianism, some sects of Hinduism, follow monotheistic belief in a God, whereas a polytheistic religion such as Hinduism holds a belief in many Gods. A popular belief at one time was that Hinduism has 330 million gods and goddesses.

While the world "Hinduism" has acquired greater currency and nomenclature, more appropriate definition centres around Vedanta philosophy or Sanatan Dharam which means an eternal ideology or system of belief that has no beginning and no end. Unlike other monotheistic religions, Vedanta believes in Advaita (Non-duality), only one God which has no second. Its multiple manifestations in the form of different gods and goddesses give an illusion of it being polytheistic in nature, but it firmly believes in the existence of only one entity-Brahman. It was never born; it does not ever die. There never was a time He was not present and indeed, there never will be a time He will not exist. He is eternal, infinite, present everywhere and attainable by everyone who seeks Him.

Science of Yoga, which is as old as God, shows several ways to attain Him. There are different words to describe this phenomenon in different religions such as Moksha, Salvation, communion, God-realisation etcetera.

Monotheistic religions largely follow the path of devotion. While some decree the traditions of idol worship, they do have symbols and some reference models to perform worship of their respective image of God. Singing hymns in a church, an image of Jesus Christ on the cross, offering daily Namaz, performing Jaap, performing Yagna to propitiate the deity are some of the classical traditions that verily are the hallmarks of devotional paradigms.

It is important to note and accept that the entire humanity is one homogeneous cohesive group of people, inhabiting the earth. They may follow different religions, different ideologies, revere different Gods, but they must necessarily converge on accepting a single power that is the creator and sustainer of the world.

Swami Vivekananda in his address at the world Parliament of religion stated that “I am proud to belong to a religion which has taught the world both tolerance and universal acceptance. We believe not only on universal toleration, but we accept all religions as true”.

He further quoted a few lines from a hymn which is repeated every day by millions of human beings. “As the different streams having their sources in different places all mingle their water in the sea, so, O Lord, the different paths which men take through different tendencies, various though they appear, crooked or straight, all lead to Thee”. This thought gets further corroboration from the concept of Vasudev Kutumbkam (वसुधैव कुटुम्बकम) that Hinduism has been propagating since many centuries.

While monotheistic religions of the world follow a set pattern of worship and religious practices, Hinduism or more correctly Vedanta offers its followers multiple choices to attain God realisation. All these practices operate under the broad umbrella of **Yoga.** The methods may be different catering to the varied strengths and sensibilities of different people, but they all take us to the same goal.

This book is an attempt to present four different paradigms of Yoga-Bhakti, Karam, Dhyan and Gyaan. Depending upon the relative strength and general propensity, the reader can make an informed choice. Journey is difficult but perseverance will make it eminently doable. At one point, they will all converge in seeking and attaining that which indeed is, only **ONE.**

The text has been embellished with interesting stories/parables to illustrate the relevance of the message incorporated. Readers will find it easy to connect with their own experiences. Science of yoga is experiential and real, as real as science can be, and a keen practitioner can validate its precepts by his own experiences.

Vinod Malhotra

Knowing and Being

One of the greatest challenges faced by mankind with respect to the spiritual tenets is not of knowing them or knowing about them, but of internalising them and practising them in real life. Every educated individual today, and their number is increasing at a much faster pace now than ever before, is in possession of a huge storehouse of knowledge. This applies to all domains. It perhaps would be more appropriate to describe what everyone knows as information. Information when processed and applied acquires the status of knowledge. But that is semantics.

To illustrate, every parent teaches a child that he should always speak the truth, that telling a lie is not a good thing. This happens at very early stages of a child's growth. The child therefore knows or is informed that he should always speak the truth. But how many can abide by this lesson throughout their life? Indeed, the parents instructing the child on the value systems (संस्कार), also find it difficult to practice what they preach. Knowing is not an issue here, but being definitely is one. Religious beliefs or spiritual tenets must manifest in our daily conduct and behaviour. It is like being a human being or being human.

In the modern era, information/knowledge has proliferated at an exponential pace and so have the means of acquiring it. Scientific and technological advancements have brought the entire humanity much closer. We seem to know everything about everything, or at least have the means to know whatever we wish to know. It is right there for everyone to access and apply. Deep inside everyone knows what is right and what is wrong. Each one of us is endowed with the power of discrimination-an important attribute of our cognitive capabilities.

The important question that must be addressed is notwithstanding all this, where do we falter and why. Why most of us are not able to put in practise what we know? Why can't we walk the talk as the expression goes?

Good standard education, religious teachings and spiritual grounding, indeed all of these put together can bring complete clarity of purpose and show us the way to a spiritual life, but that is not enough. It must manifest in whatever we think speak and act. A true definition of spirituality is the ethical manifestation of the divinity within. Axiomatically speaking, if we know it, we should do it and indeed, do it the way we know it. It should not require any extra effort. If one is spiritually enlightened, one should stop complaining, stop blaming and take whatever life throws in one's own stride. The most essential part of all this is that we should know who we really are.

There is an interesting story of a lion cub whose lioness mother died while delivering the cub. A flock of sheep was passing by, and he joined them. The lion cub grew with the sheep and did everything that a sheep would do. He ate grass, he bleated and walked at a slow pace herded by a shepherd. One fine day a big grown-up lion on a hunt, spotted the cub amid the flock and wondered what a cub was doing there following the flock and moving around happily. Finding an opportunity, he caught hold of the cub and dragged him out of the flock. The little lion started screaming and yelling what are you doing. Let me go, let me go with my flock. The big lion asked the cub to keep quiet and told him that he is a lion and not a sheep. He should not be doing what a weak animal such as a sheep does. He is a lion, mighty and strong and should be a part of the pride of lions. The cub kept screaming and remonstrating whereupon the big lion took him to a pond and told him to stand next to him and look into the water. The cub did as was asked and discovered that he and the big lion looked identical. He was then asked to roar, and the cub roared.

The cub realised his identity and started acting like a lion. He knew that he was not a sheep that he thought all the while but was a lion and thereafter acted like one. On realising that he was a lion, he did not have to do anything extra. Like the lion cub once we realise who we really are, we do not have to do anything more. We just must be what we are and act like one. We are spiritual beings who come to the world for a physical experience, and we are not physical beings who are in the world for a spiritual experience. Maya clouds our vision; we lose our identity and start bleating like a little sheep.

Our situation is little more complex than what it appears. Firstly, like the lion cub we are ignorant of our identity. We spend all our life in a state of complete ignorance. Under the spell of ignorance, we commit errors and keep doing what we should not be doing. Some wise person comes our way-like the big lion in the story above and tells us about our identity. We refuse to accept the reality, argue and often escape and go back to our comfort zone. Thankfully, the little **cub could not, and once he realised who he really was, started** behaving his real self.

Science of yoga is akin to that big lion in the story. "Know thyself "is the mantra and the science of yoga helps you to discover yourself.

CHAPTER ONE

ORIGIN OF YOGA

Yoga in everyone's life.

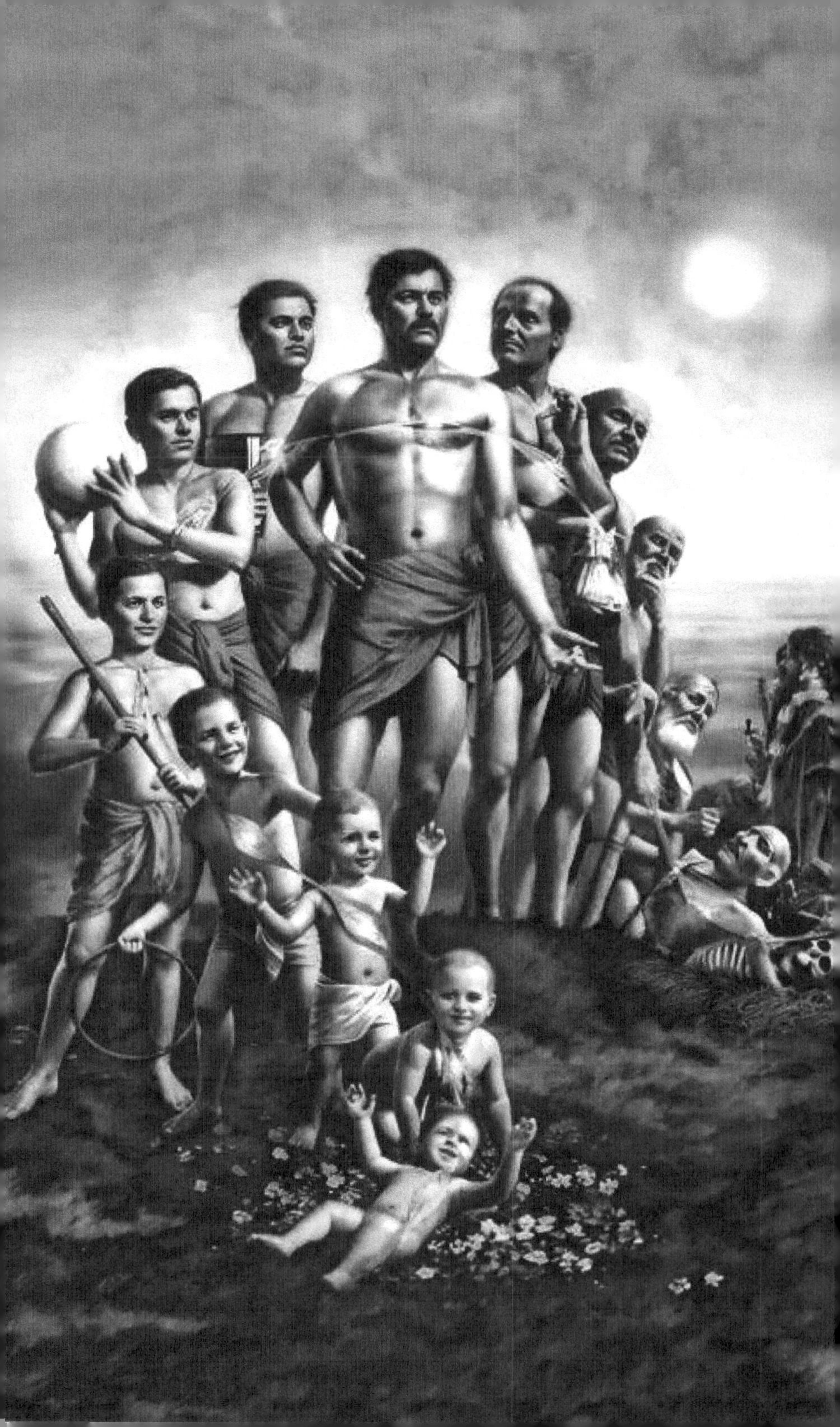

Today, Yoga is all pervading, ubiquitous and rests on the lips of every resident of our planet, regardless of nationality, colour, race, gender, belief, or ideology. Yogis, the true practitioners are rare, and rarer indeed are the ones who understand the true meaning, import, and seek adherence to its age-old and profound precepts. Science of Yoga is as old as the civilisation and many sages, enlightened people down the ages have been practising this art, re-engineered it and have greatly benefited from it, both in the spiritual and the temporal space. It covers all aspects of our journey in the world.

Our world is beautiful and possesses such diversity of living and non-living entities. Any celestial visitor would be awestruck at the creation and marvel at the ingenuity of the creator. It is extremely difficult to imagine that any independent geographical body (planet Earth), can hold variety/diversity of such vast nature in terms of humans, animals, plants on earth, air, water, and they would all co-exist in complete harmony for aeons. All creation is broadly divided into two categories-animate and inanimate. Animate or the sentient beings are quintessentially organic in nature. All living beings comprise the gross and subtle. These are born, grow, mature, decline and in fulness of time, die or wither away. Death or destruction happens to the gross, and the subtle stays in the environment in the form of an undefined component of energy, ready to move into another gross form. It reappears in a form which has no relation to the identity of its previous gross form. The cycle of birth-death-rebirth continues unabated. These are subjected to a paradigm of death, rejuvenation or revival because of their finite existential nature. Bhagwat Gita corroborates this fact in verse 28, chapter 2.

अव्यक्तादीनि भूतानि व्यक्तमध्यानि भारत ।
अव्यक्तनिधनान्येव तत्र का परिदेवना || 28 || CH 2

avyaktādīni bhūtāni vyakta-madhyāni bhārata
avyakta-nidhanānyeva tatra kā paridevanā

avyakta-ādīni—unmanifest before birth; bhūtāni—created beings; vyakta—manifest; madhyāni—in the middle; bhārata—Arjun, scion of Bharat; avyakta—unmanifest; nidhanāni—on death; eva—indeed; tatra—therefore; kā—why; paridevanā—grieve

O scion of Bharat, all created beings are unmanifest before birth, manifest in life, and again unmanifest on death. So why grieve?

Commentary

Krishna dispelled the cause of lamentation in respect to the soul in verse 2.20, and in respect to the body in verse 2.27. Now he includes both in this verse. Sage Narad instructed Yudhishthir along similar lines, in Śhrīmad Bhāgavatam: *yan manyase dhruvaṁ lokam adhruvaṁ vā na chobhayam sarvathā na hi śhochyās te snehād anyatra mohajāt* (1.13.44) [v31]

"Whether you consider the personality to be an eternal soul or to be a temporary body, or even if you accept it as an inconceivable mixture of soul and body, you should not lament in any way. The cause for lamentation is only attachment that arises out of illusion."

In the material realm, each individual soul is bound by three bodies—gross body, subtle body, causal body.

Gross body: Consists of the five gross elements of nature—earth, water, fire, air, and space.

Subtle body: Consists of eighteen elements—five life-airs, five working senses, five knowledge senses, mind, intellect, and ego.

Causal body: Consists of the account of karmas from endless past lives, including the *sanskārs* (tendencies) carried forward from previous lives.

At the time of death, the soul discards its gross body, and departs with the subtle and causal bodies. God again gives the soul another gross body according to its subtle and causal bodies and sends the soul into a suitable mother's womb for the purpose. After the soul gives up one gross body, there is a transitional phase before it receives a new gross body. This could be a few seconds in duration or a few years long. So, before birth, the soul existed with the unmanifest subtle and causal bodies. After death, it still exists in the unmanifest state. It only becomes manifest in the middle. So, death is no reason for grief.

Ashtavakra, the great sage whom King Janak took as his Guru, in chapter one of Ashtavakra Gita echoes the same truth.

साकारमनृतं विद्धि निराकारं तु निश्चलं।
एतत्तत्त्वोपदेशेन न पुनर्भवसंभव: ॥१-१८॥

आकार को असत्य जानकर निराकार को ही चिर स्थायी मानिये, इस तत्त्व को समझ लेने के बाद पुनः जन्म लेना संभव नहीं है ॥१८॥

Know that form is unreal and only the formless is permanent. Once you know this, you will not take birth again. ||18||

From unmanifest to manifest and back to an unmanifest state.

Yoga, as is evident relates to the manifest state. Human Life is to be lived, lived usefully, happily and with a clear purpose and goal. In the material context, people may have several desires for power, wealth, recognition and indeed, large multitude of humanity follows that path. However, that alone cannot be the purpose of life. In the spiritual space, the only purpose of human existence is to realise God and get out of the bondage of cycle of birth and death, and eventually unite with that ultimate reality, of which we are a part. All beliefs, all faiths the world over, accept this reality. Vedanta and many religions of the east proclaim it in the most unambiguous terms. At what stage we all got separated from that reality called God, is a subject matter of only speculation, but there is an interesting story linked to this phenomenon.

God is eternal and has always been here, and for aeons. One should not be making any guess about His age, or anything related to this. He was always there all by Himself and got bored with His perpetual unending loneliness. He wanted a way out of the boredom. God is smart and soon found a way to solve this problem. He wanted someone to play with, and created an entity called Not-God. He played to His heart content with this new friend and started enjoying the game. We all know that God is very good at whatever He does. He kept playing and soon forgot His original identity. Not-God had all the features of the God, but He was not God as everyone envisions Him to be.

That Not-God developed a distinct identity but continues to nurture a strong desire to become God all over again. We are in a way a play of God. We human beings are perennially searching for Him and that indeed, is our goal.

This is where Yoga shows the way. God realisation, though the goal of the entire humanity, without any exception is a path riddled with many difficulties. Notwithstanding, it must be pursued. However, a popular belief is that human birth is perhaps the only means to achieve that and hence, this opportunity ought not to be wasted away.

Yoga has been defined, redefined, interpreted and practised in several forms, but fundamentally, there are four paradigms that are referred to in Vedas, Upanishads, Bhagwat Gita and Patanjali Yoga Sutras. Each of these four paradigms relates to specific domains, corresponding to an individual mindset and issues that one seeks to resolve. It is possible to draw a matrix presenting these four paradigms, delineating problems, solutions and the method to solve them.

Problem	**Solution**	**Method**
1. Ignorance (Agyan)	Knowledge (Gyan)	Gyan Yoga
2. Scattered mind (Vikhshep)	Focus (Ekagrata)	Raj/Dhyan Yoga
3. Impure mind (Impurities)	Pure mind (Selflessness)	Karam Yoga
4. Lack of faith	(Worship)	Bhakti Yoga

It must be noted that while these four paradigms address different aspects of our innate nature and general inclination, each one of these methods individually, is enough to take us to our goal of God realisation. However, there exists a symbiotic relationship amongst all four forms. Hence one, or a combination of all four is recommended. For instance, Both Bhakti Yoga and Karam yoga will remove impurities of the mind. Samadhi in Raja Yoga would become easy and effortless if the mind is pure and has gone through the process of Yama, Niyama and Pratyahara. Gyan Yoga which leads to knowing the real Self, will happen only when the mind is pure and there is a clear focus developed through practice of meditation.

Yoga is as ethereal as it is ancient, and its origin can be traced to a dialogue between Krishna and Arjun in Chapter 4 of Bhagwadgita.

श्रीभगवानुवाच |
इमं विवस्वते योगं प्रोक्तवानहमव्ययम् |
विवस्वान्मनवे प्राह मनुरिक्ष्वाकवेऽब्रवीत् || 1 || CH 4

śhrī bhagavān uvācha
imaṁ vivasvate yogaṁ proktavān aham avyayam
vivasvān manave prāha manur ikṣhvākave 'bravīt

The Supreme Lord Shree Krishna said: I taught this eternal science of Yoga to the Sun God, Vivasvan, who passed it on to Manu; and Manu, in turn, instructed it to Ikshvaku.

Commentary

Merely imparting invaluable knowledge to someone is not enough. The recipients of that knowledge must appreciate its value and have faith in its authenticity. Only then will they put in the effort required to implement it practically in their lives. In this verse, Krishna establishes the credibility and importance of the spiritual wisdom he is bestowing on Arjun. Krishna informs Arjun that the knowledge being imparted unto him is not a newly created one, for the purpose of motivating him into fight the battle of Kurukshetra. It is the same eternal science of Yoga that he originally taught to Vivasvan, or Surya, Sun God, who imparted it to Manu, the original progenitor of humankind; Manu in turn taught it to Ikshvaku, first king of the Solar dynasty. This is the descending process of knowledge, where someone who is a perfect authority on the knowledge passes it down to another who wishes to know.

In contrast to this is the ascending process of acquiring knowledge, where one endeavours to enhance the frontiers of understanding through self-effort. The ascending process is laborious, imperfect, and time-consuming. For example, if we wish to learn Physics, we could either try to do it by the ascending process, where we reflect on its principles with our own intellect and then reach conclusions, or we could do it by the descending process, where we approach a good teacher of the subject. The ascending process is exceedingly time-consuming, and we may not be able to complete the inquiry in our lifetime. We also cannot be sure about the validity of our conclusions. In comparison, the descending process gives us instant access to the deepest secrets of Physics. If our teacher has perfect knowledge of Physics, then it is very straightforward—simply listen to the science from him and digest what he says. This descending process of receiving knowledge is impeccable, easy and faultless.

Every year, thousands of self-help books are released in the market, which present the authors' solutions to the problems encountered in life. These books may be helpful in a limited way, but because they are based upon the ascending process of attaining knowledge, they are imperfect. Every few years, a new theory comes along that overthrows the current ones. This ascending process is unsuitable for knowing the Absolute Truth. Divine knowledge does not need to be created by self-effort. It is the energy of God, and has existed ever since He has existed, just as heat and light are as old as the fire from which they emanate.

God and the individual soul are both eternal, and so the science of Yoga that unites the soul and God is also eternal. There is no need to speculate and formulate new theories about it. An amazing endorsement of this truism is the *Bhagavad Gita* itself, which continues to astound people with the sagacity of its perennial wisdom that remains relevant to our daily lives, even fifty centuries after it was delivered. Krishna states here that the knowledge of Yoga, which he is revealing to Arjun, is eternal and it was passed down in ancient times through the descending process, from Guru to disciple.

एवं परम्पराप्राप्तमिमं राजर्षयो विदुः ।
स कालेनेह महता योगो नष्टः परन्तप ॥ 2 ॥ CH 4

evaṁ paramparā-prāptam imaṁ rājarṣhayo viduḥ
sa kāleneha mahatā yogo naṣhṭaḥ parantapa

O subduer of enemies, the saintly kings thus received this science of Yog in a continuous tradition. But with the long passage of time, it was lost to the world.

Commentary

In the descending process of receiving divine knowledge, the disciple understands the science of God-realization from the Guru, who in turn received it from his Guru. It was in such a tradition that saintly kings like Nimi and Janak understood the science of Yog. This tradition starts from God himself, who is the first Guru of the world.

tene brahma hṛidā ya ādi-kavaye muhyanti yat sūrayaḥ (Bhāgavatam 1.1.1) [v1]

God revealed this knowledge at the beginning of creation in the heart of the first-born Brahma, and the tradition continued from him. Krishna stated in the previous verse that he also revealed this knowledge to the Sun God, Vivasvan, from whom the tradition continued as well. However, the nature of this material world is such, that with the passage of time, this knowledge got lost. Materially minded and insincere disciples interpret the teachings according to their blemished perspectives. Within a few generations, its pristine purity is contaminated. When this happens, by his causeless grace, God reestablishes the tradition for the benefit of humankind. He may do so, either by himself descending in the world, or through a great God-realized Saint, who becomes a conduit for God's work on Earth.

स एवायं मया तेऽद्य योगः प्रोक्तः पुरातनः |
भक्तोऽसि मे सखा चेति रहस्यं ह्येतदुत्तमम् || 3 || CH 4

sa evāyaṁ mayā te 'dya yogaḥ proktaḥ purātanaḥ
bhakto 'si me sakhā cheti rahasyaṁ hyetad uttamam

The same ancient knowledge of Yog, which is the supreme secret, I am today revealing unto you, because you are My friend as well as My devotee, who can understand this transcendental wisdom.

Commentary

Krishna tells Arjun that the ancient science being imparted to him is an uncommonly known secret. Secrecy in the world is maintained for two reasons: either due to selfishness in keeping the truth to oneself, or to protect the abuse of knowledge. The science of Yoga remains a secret, not for either of these reasons, but because it requires a qualification to be understood. That qualification is revealed in this verse as devotion. The deep message of the *Bhagavad Gita* is not amenable to being understood merely through scholasticism or mastery of the Sanskrit language. It requires devotion, which destroys the subtle envy of the soul toward God and enables us to accept the humble position as his tiny parts and servitors.

Arjun was a fit student of this science because he was a devotee of the Lord. Devotion to God can be practiced in any of the five sequentially higher *bhāvas*, or sentiments: 1) *Śhānt bhāv*: adoring God as our King. 2) *Dāsya bhav*: the sentiment of servitude toward God as our Master. 3) *Sakhya bhāv*: considering God as our Friend. 4) *Vātsalya bhāv*: considering God as our Child. 5) *Mādhurya bhāv*: worshipping God as our Soul-beloved. Arjun worshipped God as his Friend, and so Krishna speaks to him as his friend and devotee.

Pure heart full of devotion alone can be the true recipient of His grace. There is nothing more exalted than the knowledge of Yoga for living a life of complete fulfilment and pursuing our goal of attaining God. Arjun was Krishna's Sakha-a true friend and received His highest grace.

अर्जुन उवाच |
अपरं भवतो जन्म परं जन्म विवस्वतः |
कथमेतद्विजानीयां त्वमादौ प्रोक्तवानिति || 4 || CH 4

arjuna uvācha
aparaṁ bhavato janma paraṁ janma vivasvataḥ
katham etad vijānīyāṁ tvam ādau proktavān iti

sa evāyaṁ mayā te 'dya yogaḥ proktaḥ purātanaḥ
bhakto 'si me sakhā cheti rahasyaṁ hyetad uttamam

In verse 4, Arjuna not realising the identity of Krishna, raises a doubt about the authenticity of Krishna's assertion about His presence in the universe prior to Vivaswaan (Sun). He declares that He was present even before the world came into existence-a world that we see and perceive- the universe, galaxies, the milky way, all celestial bodies and everything tangible and intangible. Indeed, He is responsible for the creation of the world. Nothing in this universe exists without Me. In verse 39 and 42 of chapter 10 of Gita, He makes a clear proclamation to this effect.

यच्चापि सर्वभूतानां बीजं तदहमर्जुन |
न तदस्ति विना यत्स्यान्मया भूतं चराचरम् || 39 || CH 10

yach chāpi sarva-bhūtānāṁ bījaṁ tad aham arjuna
na tad asti vinā yat syān mayā bhūtaṁ charācharam

yat—which; cha—and; api—also; sarva-bhūtānām—of all living beings; bījam—generating seed; tat—that; aham—I; arjuna—Arjun; na—not; tat—that; asti—is; vinā—without; yat—which; syāt—may exist; mayā—me; bhūtam—creature; chara-acharam—moving and nonmoving

Translation

I am the generating seed of all living beings, O Arjun. No creature moving or non-moving can exist without Me.

Commentary

Krishna is both the efficient cause of all creation and the material cause. Efficient cause means that he is the creator who performs the work involved in manifesting the world. Material cause means that he is the material from which creation happens. In verses 7.10 and 9.18, Shree Krishna declared himself as “the eternal seed.” Again here, he states that he is “the generating seed.” He is stressing that he is the origin of everything, and without his potency nothing can exist.

Living beings are born in four ways: *Aṇḍaj*—born from eggs, such as birds, snakes, and lizards; *Jarāyuj*—born from the womb, such as humans, cows, dogs, and cats; *Swedaj*—born from sweat, such as lice, ticks, etc; *Udbhij*—sprouting from the earth, such as trees, creepers, grass, and corn. There are also other life forms, such as ghosts, evil spirits, manes, etc. Krishna is the origin of all of them

अथवा बहुनैतेन किं ज्ञातेन तवार्जुन |
विष्टभ्याहमिदं कृत्स्नमेकांशेन स्थितो जगत् || 42 || CH 10

atha vā bahunaitena kiṁ jñātena tavārjuna
viṣhṭabhyāham idaṁ kṛitsnam ekānśhena sthito jagat

athavā—or; bahunā—detailed; etena—by this; kim—what; jñātena tava—can be known by you; arjuna—Arjun; viṣhṭabhya—pervade and support; aham—I; idam—this; kṛitsnam—entire; eka—by one; anśhena—fraction; sthitaḥ—am situated; jagat—creation

Translation

What need is there for all this detailed knowledge, O Arjun? Simply know that by one fraction of My being, I pervade and support this entire creation.

Commentary

Krishna's statement indicates that he has already answered the question. Now, of his own accord, he wants to tell something remarkable. Having revealed many amazing aspects of his splendour, he says that the magnitude of his glory cannot be judged even from the sum of what he has described, for the entire creation of unlimited universes is held within a fraction of his being.

Why does he make a reference to a fraction of his being here? The reason is that the entire material creation consisting of unlimited universes is only one-fourth of God's entire manifestation; the remaining three-fourths is the spiritual creation.

pādo 'sya viśhwā bhūtāni tripādasyāmṛitaṁ divi
(Puruṣh Sūktam Mantra 3) [v32]

"This temporary world made from the material energy is but one part of the Supreme Divine Personality. The other three parts are his eternal abodes that are beyond the phenomenon of life and death."

Interestingly, Krishna is in front of Arjun, within the world, yet he reveals that the entire world is within a fraction of his being. This is like the story of Ganesh and Lord Shiv. Once, Sage Narad gave Lord Shiv a very special fruit. Lord Shiv's two children, Kartikeya and Ganesh both began demanding the fruit from him. Lord Shiv thought that if he would give it to any one of them, the other would think that their father was biased. So, Lord Shiv announced a competition for his two children. Whoever circumambulated the entire universe and came back to him first would get the fruit.

On hearing this, Kartikeya immediately started off to circumambulate the universe. He was athletically and powerfully built and decided to take advantage of it. In comparison, Ganesh had a plump body and felt he was handicapped in competing with his brother. So, Ganesh decided to make up for it by using his intellect. Lord Shiv and Parvati were standing there. Ganesh circumambulated them thrice, and then announced, "Father, I have done it. Please give me the fruit." Lord Shiv, "But how have you gone around the universe? You have been with us all the while." Ganesh said, "Father, you are God. The entire universe exists within you. If I have gone around you, I have gone around the entire universe." Lord Shiv had to agree that his son Ganesh was very smart, and indeed he had won the competition.

Just as Lord Shiv was standing in one place, and yet the entire world was contained in him, similarly, Krishna announces to Arjun that the entire creation, consisting of unlimited material universes, is held within a fraction of his being.

This is the loudest declaration and affirmation of the Advaita principle enshrined in the oldest scriptures of the humanity-the Vedas. There is only one without a second. Everything other than Him is His creation, His representation and just an appearance. In verse 7 of chapter 7, He gives a beautiful illustration of every entity in the universe as beads strung in a single thread.

मत्तः परतरं नान्यत्किञ्चिदस्ति धनञ्जय |
मयि सर्वमिदं प्रोतं सूत्रे मणिगणा इव || 7 || CH 7

mattaḥ—than me; para-taram—superior; na—not; anyat kiñchit—anything else; asti—there is; dhanañjaya—Arjun, conqueror of wealth; mayi—in me; sarvam—all; idam—which we see; protam—is strung; sūtre—on a thread; maṇi-gaṇāḥ—beads; iva—like

Translation

There is nothing higher than Myself, O Arjun. Everything rests in Me, as beads strung on a thread.

Commentary

Here, Krishna states about His dominion and His Supreme position in this universe. He is the Substratum over which this entire creation exists; He is the Creator, Sustainer, and Annihilator. Like the beads strung in a thread, which can move in their place, God has given individual souls the free will to act as they wish, yet their existence is bound to Him. The Śhwetāśhvatar Upaniṣhad states:

na tatsamaśhchābhyadhikaśhcha dṛiśhyate
parāsya śhaktirvividhaiva śhrūyate (6.8)

"There is nothing equal to God, nor is there anything superior to Him." As the first-born Brahma prays to Krishna:

īśhwaraḥ paramaḥ kṛiṣhṇaḥ sachchidānanda vigrahaḥ
*anādirādir govindaḥ sarva kārana kāraṇam (*Brahma Samhitā 5.1)

"Krishna is the Supreme Lord, who is eternal, omniscient, and infinite bliss. He is without beginning and end, the origin of all, and the cause of all causes."

Going further, Krishna, vide two verses 7 & 8 of chapter 4, that have become the iconic verses of Gita, declares the purpose of his incarnation in human forms.

यदा यदा हि धर्मस्य ग्लानिर्भवति भारत |
अभ्युत्थानमधर्मस्य तदात्मानं सृजाम्यहम् || 7 || CH 4

yadā yadā hi dharmasya glānir bhavati bhārata
abhyutthānam adharmasya tadātmānaṁ sṛijāmyaham

yadā yadā—whenever; hi—certainly; dharmasya—of righteousness; glāniḥ—decline; bhavati—is; bhārata—Arjun, descendant of Bharat; abhyutthānam—increase; adharmasya—of unrighteousness; tadā—at that time; ātmānam—self; sṛijāmi—manifest; aham—I

Whenever there is a decline in righteousness and an increase in unrighteousness, O Arjun, at that time I manifest Myself on earth.

Commentary

Dharma is verily the prescribed actions that are conducive to our spiritual growth and progress; the reverse of this is *adharma* (unrighteousness). When unrighteousness prevails, the creator and administrator of the world intervenes by descending and reestablishing *dharma*. Such a descension of God is called an *Avatār*. The word "Avatar" has been adopted from Sanskrit into English and is commonly used for people's images on the media screen. In this text, we will be using it in its original Sanskrit connotation, to refer to the divine descension of God. Twenty-four such descensions have been listed in the Śhrīmad Bhāgavatam. However, the Vedic scriptures state that there are innumerable descensions of God:

janma-karmābhidhānāni santi me 'ṅga sahasraśhaḥ
na śhakyante 'nusaṅkhyātum anantatvān mayāpi hi
(Bhāgavatam 10.51.37) [v5]

"Nobody can count the infinite Avatars of God since the beginning of eternity." These Avatars are classified in four categories, as stated below:

1. *Āveśhāvatār*—when God manifests his special powers in an individual soul and acts through him. The sage Narad is an example of *Āveśhāvatār*. The Buddha is also an example of *Āveśhāvatār*.

2. *Prābhavāvatār*—these are the descensions of God in the personal form, where he displays some of his divine powers. *Prābhavāvatārs* are also of two kinds:

    a) Where God reveals himself only for a few moments, completes his work, and then departs. Hansavatar is an example of this, where God manifested before the Kumaras, answered their question, and left.
    b) Where the Avatar remains on the earth for many years. Ved Vyas, who wrote the eighteen Puranas and the Mahabharat, and divided the Vedas into four parts, is an example of such an Avatar.

3. *Vaibhavatār*—when God descends in his divine form, and manifests more of his divine powers. Matsyavatar, Kurmavatar, Varahavatar are all examples of *Vaibhavatārs*.

4. *Parāvasthāvatār*—when God manifests all his divine powers in his personal divine form. Shree Krishna, Shree Ram, and Nrisinghavatar are all *Parāvasthāvatār*.

This classification does not imply that any one *Avatār* is bigger than the other. Ved Vyas, who is himself an *Avatār*, clearly states this: *sarve pūrṇāḥ śhāśhvatāśhcha dehāstasya paramātmanaḥ* (Padma Purāṇ)[v6]

"All the descensions of God are replete with all divine powers; they are all perfect and complete." Hence, we should not differentiate one Avatar as bigger and another as smaller. However, in each descension, God manifests his powers based on the objectives he wishes to accomplish during that descension. The remaining powers reside latently within the Avatar. Hence, the above classifications were created.

परित्राणाय साधूनां विनाशाय च दुष्कृताम् |
धर्मसंस्थापनार्थाय सम्भवामि युगे युगे || 8 ||

paritrāṇāya sādhūnāṁ vināśhāya cha duṣhkṛitām
dharma-sansthāpanārthāya sambhavāmi yuge yuge

To protect the righteous, to annihilate the evil, and to reestablish the principles of dharma I appear on this earth, in different time zones.

Commentary

Having stated in the last verse that God descends in the world, he now states the three reasons for doing so:

1) To annihilate the wicked.
2) To protect the pious.
3) To establish dharma. However, if we closely study these three points, none of the three reasons seem very convincing:

To protect the righteous. God is seated in the hearts of his devotees, and always protects them from within. There is no need to take an Avatar for this purpose.

To annihilate the wicked. God is all-powerful and can kill the wicked merely by wishing it. Why should he have to take an Avatar to accomplish this?

To establish dharma. Dharma is eternally described in the Vedas. God can reestablish it through a Saint; he does not need to descend himself, in his personal form, to accomplish this.
How then do we make sense of the reasons that have been stated in this verse? Let's delve a little deeper to grasp the import of what Krishna is stating.
The biggest dharma that the soul can engage in is devotion to God. That is what God facilitates by taking an *Avatār*. When God descends in the world, he reveals his divine forms, names, virtues, pastimes, abodes, and associates. This provides the souls with an easy basis for devotion. Since the mind needs a form to focus upon and to connect with, the formless aspect of God is very difficult to worship. On the other hand, devotion to the personal form of God is easy for people to comprehend, simple to perform, and sweet to engage in.

Krishna, aware of a deep-seated sense of unease experienced by most of the mankind for whom identification with something unmanifest is difficult, makes the following statement.

क्लेशोऽधिकतरस्तेषामव्यक्तासक्तचेतसाम् ||
अव्यक्ता हि गतिर्दुःखं देहवद्भिरवाप्यते || 5 || CH 12

kleśho 'dhikataras teṣhām avyaktāsakta-chetasām
avyaktā hi gatir duḥkhaṁ dehavadbhir avāpyate

kleśhaḥ—tribulations; adhika-taraḥ—full of; teṣhām—of those; avyakta—to the unmanifest; āsakta—attached; chetasām—whose minds; avyaktā—the unmanifest; hi—indeed; gatiḥ—path; duḥkham—exceedingly difficult; deha-vadbhiḥ—for the embodied; avāpyate—is reached

Translation

For those whose minds are attached to the unmanifest, the path of realization is full of tribulations. Worship of the unmanifest is exceedingly difficult for embodied beings.

Commentary

Having embraced worshippers of all His various manifestations into the fold, Krishna again reiterates His preference for the worship of the personal form. He surmises the worship of the impersonal Brahman by saying that it is an exceedingly challenging path that is full of tribulations.

Why is the worship of the formless Brahman so difficult? The first and foremost reason for this is that we humans possess a form ourselves and we have been habituated to interact with forms in endless lifetimes. Thus, in our pursuit of love of God, if our mind has a form to meditate upon, it becomes easy to focus and increase our attachment to the Lord. However, in the case of the formless, the intellect cannot conceive of it, and the mind and senses have no tangible object to relate to. So, our endeavours of meditating on God and fixing the mind's attachment to Him become difficult.

Worship of Brahman is also difficult in comparison to that of *Bhagavān* for another reason. The difference in paths can be understood through the *markaṭ-kiśhore nyāya* (the logic of the baby) monkey, and *mārjār-kiśhore nyāya* (the logic of the baby kitten). The baby monkey is responsible for holding onto her mother's stomach; it is not helped by its mother. When the mother monkey jumps from one branch to another, the onus of clinging tightly onto the mother is upon the baby, and if it is unable to do so, it falls. In contrast, a kitten is very small and delicate, but the mother takes the responsibility of transporting it from one place to another, by holding the kitten from behind the neck and lifting it up. In this analogy, the devotees of the formless can be compared to the baby monkey and the devotees of the personal form can be compared to the baby kitten. Those who worship the formless Brahman have the onus of progressing on the path by themselves, because Brahman does not bestow grace upon them. Brahman is not only formless, but also without attributes. It has been described as nirguṇa (without qualities), nirviśheṣh (without attributes), and nirākār (without form). From this, it follows that Brahman does not manifest the quality of grace. The jñānīs who worship God as nirguṇa, nirviśheṣh, and nirākār, must rely entirely upon self-effort for progress. On the other hand, the personal form of God is an ocean of compassion and mercy. Hence, devotees of the personal form receive the help of divine support in their sādhanā. Based on the protection that God bestows upon His devotees, Krishna stated in verse 9.31: "O son of Kunti, declare it boldly that no devotee of Mine is ever lost."

Thus, since the descension of Lord Krishna 5,000 years ago, billions of souls have made his divine *Leela* (pastimes) as the basis of their devotion and purified their minds with ease and joy. Similarly, the Ramayana has provided the souls with a popular basis for devotion for innumerable centuries. When the TV show, Ramayana, first began airing on Indian national television on Sunday mornings, all the streets of India would become empty. The pastimes of Lord Ram held such fascination for the people that they would be glued to their television sets to see the *Leela* on the screen. This reveals how Lord Ram's descension provided the basis for devotion to billions of souls in history. The Ramayana says:

rām eka tāpasa tiya tārī, nāma koṭi khala kumati sudhārī [v7]

"In his descension period, Lord Ram helped only one Ahalya (Sage Gautam's wife, whom Ram released from the body of stone). However, since then, by chanting the divine name "Ram," billions of fallen souls have elevated themselves." So, a deeper understanding of this verse is:

To establish dharma: God descends to establish the dharma of devotion by providing souls with his names, forms, pastimes, virtues, abodes, and associates, with the help of which they may engage in *bhakti* and purify their minds.

To kill the wicked: Along with God, to help facilitate his divine pastimes, some liberated Saints descend and pretend to be miscreants. For example, Ravan and Kumbhakarna were Jaya and Vijaya who descended from the divine abode of God. They pretended to be demons and opposed and fought with Ram. They could not have been killed by anyone else, since they were divine personalities. So, God slayed such demons as a part of his *Leela*. And having killed them, he sent them to his divine abode, since that was where they came from in the first place.

To protect the righteous: Many souls had become sufficiently elevated in their *sadhana* (spiritual practice) to qualify to meet God face-to-face. When Krishna descended in the world, these eligible souls got their first opportunity to participate in God's divine pastimes. For example, some *gopīs* (cowherd women of Vrindavan, where Shree Krishna manifested his pastimes) were liberated souls who had descended from the divine abode to assist in Shree Krishna's *Leela*. Other *gopīs* were materially bound souls who got their first chance to meet and serve God and participate in his *Leela*. So, when Shree Krishna descended in the world, such qualified souls got the opportunity to perfect their devotion by directly participating in the pastimes of God.

This is the deeper meaning of the verse. However, it is not wrong if someone wishes to cognize the verse more literally or metaphorically.

While the science of yoga has been delivered to the world in several names and dimensions, basically, two forms have been recognized and practised somewhat, world-wide. These are, Karam yoga and Raja yoga. Indeed, a large multitude of the mankind associates Gita with the philosophy of Karam yoga- very few though practise it truly in life. Raja yoga, also known as Dhyana yoga, is practised to achieve a state of mediation through asanas and pranayama, but its methods and essence are not easily comprehended, much less observed with purity and self-discipline. In the physical-centred world, yoga which is quintessentially metaphysical, several essential features other than emphasis on physical fitness, have been largely ignored. Both Dhyan Yoga and Karam Yoga require an affirmative action. Practitioners must perform certain actions with a complete sense of detachment from the material world or stay engaged in meditational state by bringing one's mind and intellect to concentrate on the image of God. Raja Yoga requires complete cessation of all worldly modifications.

There are other two contrasting paradigms-Bhakti Yoga and Gyan Yoga. Here there is no overt action as such. These are purely devotion-centred, or realisation driven. You are not called upon to do anything. You just must surrender to Him in absolute devotion or realise your true self.

The objective of writing this book is to take the reader on a journey of several forms of yoga practices, which constitute the foundational platform of knowledge, self-discipline, happy and productive living, and ultimate enlightenment.

In the following pages, different aspects of four paradigms of Yoga will be discussed. These are.

Bhakti Yoga-Foundational yoga with faith and devotion as the main instruments. If there is a lack of faith, you practise Bhakti Yoga.

Karam Yoga-Detachment and selflessness. Absolute focus on work without being burdened with the reward, you take to Karam Yoga.

Raja Yoga-Meditation in achieving stillness of mind. To bring about calmness to a mind which is disturbed with numerous thoughts, Raja Yoga or Dhyana Yoga is recommended. This is also known as Ashtanga Yoga.

Gyan Yoga-Realization of truth and ultimate reality. We are all deluded by ignorance about Self, the world by Maya. Gyan Yoga is the remedy.

While delivering the most profound message of Bhagwat Gita during the battlefield of Mahabharata, Krishna advises Arjuna to be always a yogi.

नैते सृती पार्थ जानन्योगी मुह्यति कश्चन ।
तस्मात्सर्वेषु कालेषु योगयुक्तो भवार्जुन || 27 || CH 8

naite sṛitī pārtha jānan yogī muhyati kaśhchana
tasmāt sarveṣhu kāleṣhu yoga-yukto bhavārjuna

na—never; ete—these two; sṛitī—paths; pārtha—Arjun, the son of Pritha; jānan—knowing; yogī—a yogi; muhyati—bewildered; kaśhchana—any; tasmāt—therefore; sarveṣhu kāleṣhu—always; yoga-yuktaḥ—situated in Yog; bhava—be; arjuna—Arjun

Yogis who know the secret of these two paths, O Parth, are never bewildered. Therefore, always remain situated in Yoga (union with God).

Those relentless souls who strive for *Yog* or union with God are true yogis. They recognize themselves to be tiny fragments of God and His eternal beatitude. They also realize the temporary nature of the material world and the futility of a materialistic life. Therefore, instead of running behind sensual pleasures, they endeavour to enhance their love for God. Such souls are on the path of eternal light.

On the other hand, are the ignorant souls, who are under the influence of maya, the material energy. They recognize themselves as only the body and the material world around them as the source of their pleasure. They continue to live through the miseries of material existence, being disdainful toward God or His eternal opulence. Thus, such souls are on the path of perpetual darkness.

In this verse, Krishna urges Arjun to recognize the difference between these two paths and choose the path of light, thus become a yogi. It is not that many of us do not take the path of light, but after some times are back on the path of darkness.

For instance, someone wishes to go east and walks one mile toward the rising sun in the morning. He rests in the afternoon for a while. Then he starts walking again toward the sun, which is now in the west. He walks for two miles only to find in the evening that he is one mile farther in the west from where he had started. Similarly, treading on the path of light only for some time will not work; it needs to be a constant process, else one will slip back into darkness again. Therefore, in this verse Krishna adds the phrase, "at all times." It is for us to recognize the importance of being always a yogi. And avoid the danger of sliding back into the path of darkness.

तपस्विभ्योऽधिकोयोगी
ज्ञानिभ्योऽपिमतोऽधिकः।
कर्मिभ्यश्चाधिकोयोगी
तस्माद्योगीभवार्जुन || 43 || CH 6

tapasvibhyo 'dhiko yogī
jñānibhyo 'pi mato 'dhikaḥ
karmibhyaśh chādhiko yogī
tasmād yogī bhavārjuna

tapasvibhyaḥ—than the ascetics; adhikaḥ—superior; yogī—a yogi; jñānibhyaḥ—than the persons of learning; api—even; mataḥ—considered; adhikaḥ—superior; karmibhyaḥ—than the ritualistic performers; cha—and; adhikaḥ—superior; yogī—a yogi; tasmāt—therefore; yogī—a yogi; bhava—just become; arjuna—Arjun

A yogi is superior to the *tapasvī* (ascetic), superior to the *jñānī* (a person of learning), and even superior to the *karmī* (ritualistic performer). Therefore, O Arjun, strive to be a yogi.

A *tapasvī* (ascetic) is one who accepts voluntary mortification and lives an extremely austere lifestyle, refraining from sensual pleasures and the accumulation of material wealth, as an aid in the pursuit of salvation. A *jñānī* is a person of learning who actively engages in the cultivation of knowledge. A *karmī* is one who performs the Vedic rituals for attaining material opulence and the celestial abodes. Shree Krishna declares the yogi to be superior to them all. The reason for this is simple. The goal of the *karmī, jñānī,* and *tapasvī* is worldly attainment; they are still at the bodily platform of existence. The yogi is striving not for the world, but for God. As a result, the yogi's accomplishment is at the spiritual platform and is superior to them all.

While for a person already on a spiritual path, Yoga helps him to pursue his goal of enlightenment, and for the ordinary mortal like us, Yoga shows a way out of suffering that we are subjected to during our journey of life. The world, Samsara is another name of suffering and while moments of happiness are few and far between, suffering knocks at doorsteps almost incessantly. Buddha realised this early in life. Legend has it that at the age of 29, Prince Siddartha Gautama was completely shaken by the "Four Signs" he saw in succession; an old man, a sick person, a corpse being carried to cremation, and a monk in meditation beneath a tree. Gautama later became the man known as Buddha when he decided to renounce the empire and started leading a life of an ascetic.

Mahatma Buddha established four noble Truths, and these are.

1. Dukkha, ill being.
2. Samudaya, the origination of ill being.
3. Nirodh, the cessation or annihilation of suffering
4. Marga, the path to the cessation of suffering.

Every living being in the world is subjected to a constant stream of happiness and misery, much of it is our own making. We are perennially engaged in the performance of various actions. Our thoughts, speech and actions that constitute the body of our Karma, inevitably lead to certain consequences. We get into a bondage of attachment, desires and in directionless pursuit of material pleasures.

The science of Yoga, if understood and practised properly is eminently designed to take us on the path of cessation of suffering. Dukh and Sukh will happen, they will come and go, and Yoga will give us the strength and sagacity to bear them, make us realise our real self and help us on the path of enlightenment-the goal of the entire mankind.

सुखदु:खे समे कृत्वा लाभालाभौ जयाजयौ |
ततो युद्धाय युज्यस्व नैवं पापमवाप्स्यसि || 38 || CH 2

sukha-duḥkhe same kṛitvā lābhālābhau jayājayau
tato yuddhāya yujyasva naivaṁ pāpam avāpsyasi

sukha—happiness; duḥkhe—in distress; same kṛitvā—treating alike; lābha-alābhau—gain and loss; jaya-ajayau—victory and defeat; tataḥ—thereafter; yuddhāya—for fighting; yujyasva—engage; na—never; evam—thus; pāpam—sin; avāpsyasi—shall incur

Translation

Fight for the sake of duty, treating alike happiness and distress, loss and gain, victory and defeat. Fulfilling your responsibility in this way, you will never incur sin.

Commentary

Having motivated Arjun from the mundane level, Shree Krishna now moves deeper into the science of work. Arjun had expressed his fear that by killing his enemies he would incur sin. Shree Krishna addresses this apprehension. He advises Arjun to do his duty, without attachment to the fruits of his actions. Such an attitude to work will release him from any sinful reactions.

When we work with selfish motives, we create karmas, which bring about their subsequent karmic reactions. The Māṭhar Śhruti states:

puṇyena puṇya lokaṁ nayati pāpena pāpamubhābhyāmeva manuṣhyalokam [v34]

"If you do good deeds, you will go to the celestial abodes; if you do bad deeds, you will go to the nether regions; if you do a mixture of both, you will come back to the planet Earth." In either case, we get bound by the reactions of our karmas. Thus, mundane good deeds are also binding. They result in material rewards, which add to the stockpile of our karmas and thicken the illusion that there is happiness in the world.

However, if we give up selfish motives, then our actions no longer create any karmic reactions. For example, murder is a sin, and the judicial law of every country of the world declares it to be a punishable offence. But if a policeman in the discharge of his duty kills the leader of a gang of bandits, he is not punished for it. If a soldier kills an enemy soldier in battle, he is not punished for it. In fact, he can even be awarded a medal for bravery. The reason for apparent lack of punishment is that these actions are not motivated by any ill-will or personal motive; they are performed as a matter of duty to the country. God's law is quite similar. If one gives up all selfish motives and works merely for the sake of duty toward the Supreme, such work does not create any karmic reactions.

So, Krishna advises Arjun to become detached from outcomes and simply focus on doing his duty. When he fights with the attitude of equanimity, treating victory and defeat, pleasure and pain as the same, then despite killing his enemies, he will never incur sin. This subject is also repeated later in the *Bhagavad Gita*, in verse 5.10: "Just as a lotus leaf is untouched by water, those who dedicate all their actions to God, abandoning all attachment, remain untouched by sin."

All forms of Yoga confer equanimity, sagacity and keep one spiritually grounded. One achieves peace, equilibrium unaffected by the sufferings of the world and eventually acquire a state of bliss.

यं लब्ध्वा चापरं लाभं मन्यते नाधिकं ततः |
यस्मिन्स्थितो न दुःखेन गुरुणापि विचाल्यते || 22 || CH 6

yaṁ labdhvā chāparaṁ lābhaṁ manyate nādhikaṁ tataḥ
yasmin sthito na duḥkhena guruṇāpi vichālyate

yam—which; labdhvā—having gained; cha—and; aparam—any other; lābham—gain; manyate—considers; na—not; adhikam—greater; tataḥ—than that; yasmin—in which; sthitaḥ—being situated; na—never; duḥkhena—by sorrow; guruṇā—(by) the greatest; api—even; vichālyate—is shaken

Translation

Having gained that state, one does not consider any attainment to be greater. Being thus established, one is not shaken even amid the greatest calamity.

Commentary

In the material realm, no extent of attainment satiates a person totally. A poor person strives hard to become rich and feels satisfied if he or she is able to become a millionaire. But when that same millionaire looks at a billionaire, discontentment sets in again. The billionaire is also discontented by looking at an even richer person. No matter what happiness we get, when we perceive a higher state of happiness, the feeling of unfulfillment lingers. But happiness achieved from the state of Yog is the infinite bliss of God. Since there is nothing higher than that, on experiencing that infinite bliss, the soul naturally perceives that it has reached its goal.

God's divine bliss is also eternal, and it can never be snatched away from the yogi who has attained it once. Such a God-realized soul, though residing in the material body, remains in the state of divine consciousness. Sometimes, externally, it seems that the Saint is facing tribulations in the form of illness, antagonistic people, and oppressive environment, but internally the Saint retains divine consciousness and continues to relish the bliss of God. Thus, even the biggest difficulty cannot shake such a Saint. Established in union with God, the Saint rises above bodily consciousness and is thus not affected by bodily harm. Accordingly, we hear from the Puranas how Prahlad was put in a pit of snakes, tortured with weapons, placed in the fire, thrown off a cliff, etc. but none of these difficulties could break Prahlad's devotional union with God.

As a final verdict on the benefits of yoga, Krishna declares that having attained the state of yoga nothing is more attainable. Even the most difficult calamity cannot disturb the yogi. He transcends all desires and becomes immune to all sufferings.

CHAPTER TWO

BHAKTI YOGA

Yoga in everyone's life.

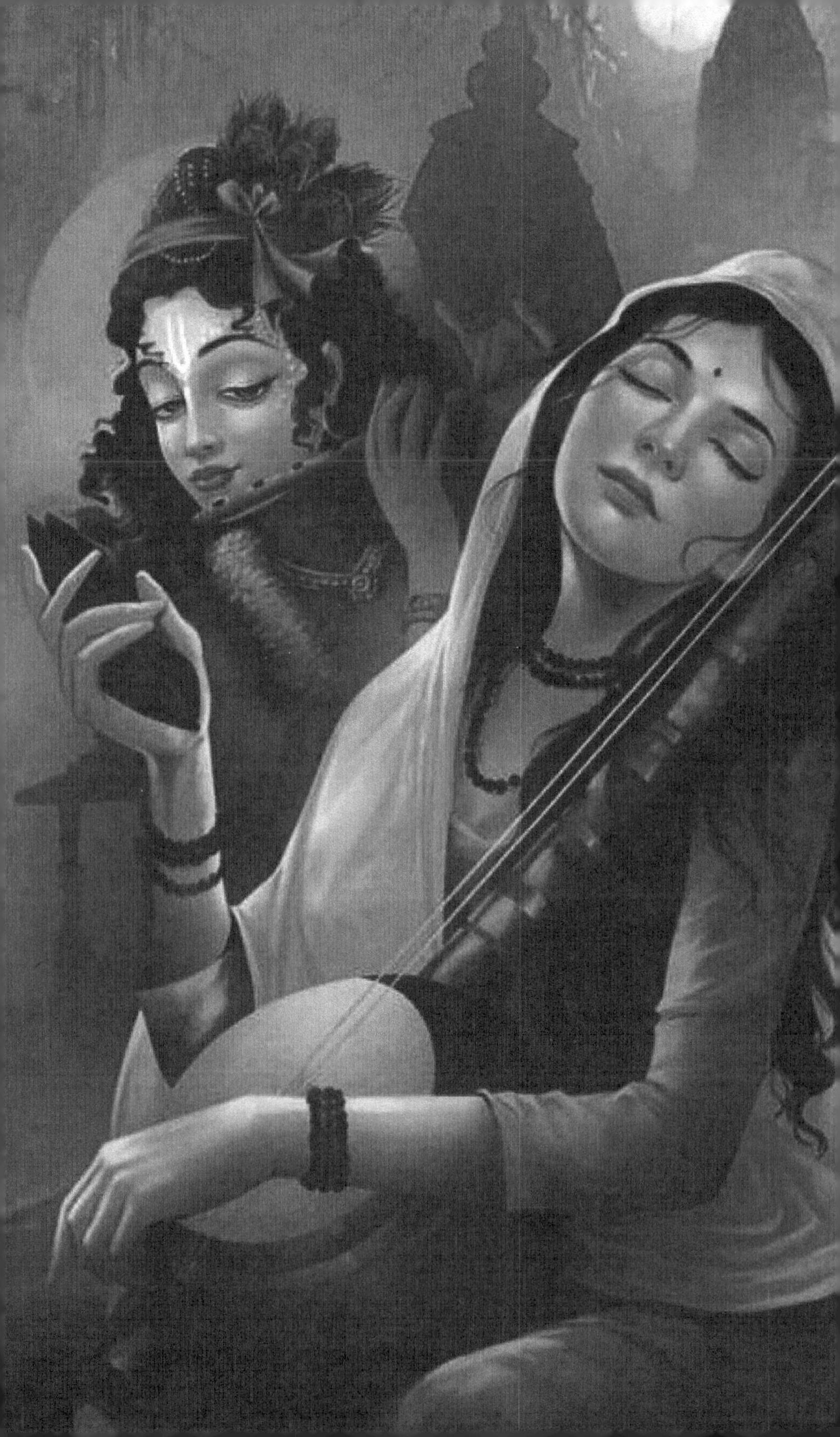

BHAKTIYOGA

The word '**Yoga**' has been derived from the Sanskrit root **'Yuj'** which means to join, or to yoke or to unite.

It also means "to become one with". Concept of yoga is strictly in line with the recognition of classical 'Advaitvad' (Non-duality) principle propounded in the ancient texts of Vedas. Non-duality literally means 'One' that has no second. Yoga therefore creates a path or several paths, where an individual self loses his identity and joins the Supreme consciousness of which he/she is an integral part. By that he becomes one with Him, the ultimate reality which always was, is and will be. By that he realizes the truth and his own identity.

Of all forms of yoga currently in vogue, the easiest and the most powerful medium to reach the goal is 'Bhakti Yoga'-the path of devotion, surrender, "Samarpan" to that Supreme consciousness. There are some remarkable features of this practice, not found in other forms.

1. It is easy to practice.
2. It is available to everyone in the world.
3. It does not need any pre-qualifications.
4. It does not impose any social barriers.
5. It can be practised anytime anywhere.
6. There is complete freedom to choose the subject/object of your devotion.
7. This practice does not require any external support.
8. It only needs faith in the existence of One supreme power.
9. It has the potential to convert an atheist to a theist.
10. It is perhaps the only form of Yoga which is practised by all, regardless of the religion or ideology they follow.
11. It really forms the foundation of all forms of yoga practised anywhere in the world.
12. Bhakti yoga heralds the journey of an individual to higher forms, and with absolute devotion and surrender to the deity of his choice, he achieves peace and bliss. This alone helps him to realise the truth and his own identity.

Bhakti yoga is simple, uncomplicated and straightforward and just needs a combination of love and faith. Love is basic and a standard emotion, everyone experiences in his life, indeed several times and with multiple beings and objects during one's lifetime. This is what keeps everyone bound, connected- from a smallest living being in the animal world to the highest creation of nature-human beings. In a classic mode it refers to a feeling of deep emotional connect between two persons, or with more, such as relations, friends and people we meet up during our journey of life.

Sometimes it takes an extreme form where two persons in love seem, to pledge a lifelong attachment and consider that as the main purpose of their existence. There is nothing amiss in it, but attachment of this nature often becomes a cause of deep anguish and misery.

Bhakti yoga transcends these limitations and gives an experience of love for the entire mankind. Through this, you experience God in every creation and become one with everyone. In every entity, animate or inanimate you only see Him. Indeed, in everyone and in everything you see only your own reflection as a representation of God. Love of this nature is sans any worldly attachments.

राम ही राम में सब जग जानु

Meerabai, Surdas, Chaitanya Maha Prabhu were great examples of the bhakti yoga at its Zenith. They saw none other than the persona of Krishna in all states- awake, dream and even during deep sleep. In fact, in bhakti yoga, you become one with your 'Isht', (इष्ट) and any distinction between the devotee and the subject of his devotion ceases to exist. Bhakti yoga forms an unbreakable bond between the devotee and God in the form of a personal God, often referred as (ईश्वर.)

The concept of bhakti emanates from an innate and essential nature of all beings. Human beings are an absolute personification of faith and trust. Krishna in verse 3, chapter 17 explains this.

सत्त्वानुरूपा सर्वस्य श्रद्धा भवति भारत |
श्रद्धामयोऽयं पुरुषो यो यच्छ्रद्धः स एव सः || 3 || CH 17

sattvānurūpā sarvasya śhraddhā bhavati bhārata
śhraddhā-mayo 'yaṁ puruṣho yo yach-chhraddhaḥ sa eva saḥ

sattva-anurūpā—conforming to the nature of one's mind; sarvasya—all; śhraddhā—faith; bhavati—is; bhārata—Arjun, the scion of Bharat; śhraddhāmayaḥ—possessing faith; ayam—that; puruṣhaḥ—human being; yaḥ—who; yat-śhraddhaḥ—whatever the nature of their faith; saḥ—their; eva—verily; saḥ—they

Translation

The faith of all humans conforms to the nature of their mind. All people possess faith, and whatever the nature of their faith, that is verily what they are.

Commentary

As a standard practice, we all repose our faith somewhere or the other. Where we decide to place our faith and what we choose to believe in, practically shapes the direction of our life. Those who develop the conviction that money is of paramount importance in the world spend their entire life accumulating it. Those who believe that fame counts more than anything else dedicate their time and energy in chasing political positions and social designations. Those who believe in noble values, sacrifice everything to uphold them. Mahatma Gandhi had faith in the incomparable importance of *satya* (truth) and *ahinsā* (non-violence), and by the strength of his convictions he launched a non-violent movement that succeeded in evicting from India the most powerful empire in the world. Those who develop deep faith in the overriding importance of God-realization renounce their material life in search of him. Thus, Krishna states that the quality of our faith decides the direction of our life. In turn, the quality of our faith is decided by the nature of our mind.

Bhakti is also a stepping platform for Gyan yoga. Acquisition of knowledge (Gyan) must necessarily be preceded by immersion in complete faith and control of senses and sense gratification. A person without the strength of faith, wanders around in wilderness and is never at peace with self or the environment.

श्रद्धावान् लभते ज्ञानं तत्परः संयतेन्द्रियः |
ज्ञानं लब्ध्वा परां शान्तिमचिरेणाधिगच्छति || 39 || CH 4

śhraddhāvān—a faithful person; labhate—achieves; jñānam—divine knowledge; tat-paraḥ—devoted (to that); sanyata—controlled; indriyaḥ—senses; jñānam—transcendental knowledge; labdhvā—having achieved; parām—supreme; śhāntim—peace; achireṇa—without delay; adhigachchhati—attains

Translation

Those whose faith is deep and who have practiced controlling their mind and senses attain divine knowledge. Through such transcendental knowledge, they quickly attain everlasting supreme peace.

Commentary

Krishna now introduces the concept of faith in the context of knowledge. Not all spiritual truths are immediately perceptible; some of them can only be experienced after having attained sufficient elevation on the path. If we only accept what we can presently verify or comprehend, we will be bereft of the higher spiritual secrets. Faith helps us accept what we cannot understand at present. Jagadguru Shankaracharya has defined faith as follows:

guru vedānta vākyeṣhu dṛiḍho viśhvāsaḥ śhraddhā [v37]

"Faith means firm confidence in the words of the Guru and the scriptures." When such faith is placed upon a wrong personality, it can lead to disastrous consequences. But when it is placed on the true Guru, it opens the pathway for eternal welfare.

However, blind faith is not a desirable thing. Before placing it on any Guru, we must use our intellect to confirm that the Guru has realized the Absolute Truth, and he is teaching it in accordance with the eternal Vedic scriptures. Once this is confirmed, then we should strive to deepen our faith in such a Guru and surrender to God under his guidance.

The Shvetashvatar Upaniṣhad states:

yasya deve parā bhaktir yathā deve tathā gurau
tasyaite kathitā hyarthāḥ prakāśhante mahātmanaḥ
(6.23) [v38]

"The imports of all the Vedic knowledge are revealed within the hearts of those who engage with unflinching faith in devotion toward Guru and God."

अज्ञश्चाश्रद्दधानश्च संशयात्मा विनश्यति |
नायं लोकोऽस्ति न परो न सुखं संशयात्मन: || 40 || CH 4

ajñaḥ—the ignorant; cha—and; aśhraddadhānaḥ—without faith; cha—and; sanśhaya—skeptical; ātmā—a person; vinaśhyati—falls down; na—never; ayam—in this; lokaḥ—world; asti—is; na—not; paraḥ—in the next; na—not; sukham—happiness; sanśhaya-ātmanaḥ—for the skeptical soul

Translation

But persons who possess neither faith nor knowledge, and who are of a doubting nature, suffer a downfall. For the sceptical souls, there is no happiness either in this world or the next.

Commentary

The Bhakti Rasāmṛit Sindhu classifies sādhaks into three classes based on the degree of faith and knowledge:

śhāstre yuktau cha nipuṇaḥ sarvathā ḍriḍha-niśhchayaḥ
prauḍha-śhraddho 'dhikārī yaḥ sa bhaktāvuttamo mataḥ
yaḥ śhāstrādiṣhvanipuṇaḥ śhraddhāvān sa tu madhyamaḥ
yo bhavet komala śhraddhaḥ sa kaniṣhṭho nigadyate (1.2.17-19) [v39]

"The highest Sadhak (spiritual aspirant) is one who possesses knowledge of the scriptures and is also endowed with firm faith. The medium class Sadhak is one who does not have knowledge of the scriptures but is endowed with faith toward God and Guru. The lowest class Sadhak is one, who neither has scriptural knowledge nor is endowed with faith." For the third category, Krishna says that such persons cannot attain peace either in this life or hereafter.

Even worldly activities require the exercise of faith. For example, if a person goes to a restaurant and places an order for the meal, he has faith that the restaurant will not serve food that is stale or contaminated. If, however, he is besieged with doubts and wants to subject every food item to a chemical test first, how will he ever enjoy the meal? Similarly, a man goes to barber shop to get a shave and sits on the chair while the barber moves the sharp edge of his knife over his throat. Now, if the man doubts the barber and suspects his having an intention of harming him, he will not be able to sit still. Hence, Krishna says in this verse that for the doubting person there is no happiness either in this world or in the next. Much of the transactions in the business world, where huge amount of money is involved happen because of faith and trust. However, it is always advisable to exercise due caution and diligence before resorting to faith where stakes are very high.

History is replete with examples of devotion or bhakti yoga, leading to immense knowledge and wisdom that is eternal and relevant in all situations. Valmiki, a dacoit who robbed and killed without a thought, became a great devotee of Ram and went on to create one of the greatest classics of Indian mythology-Ramayana. All subsequent versions of the story of Ram drew their authenticity from Valmiki's work.

Kabir, a poor illiterate weaver created poetic works of epic proportions, encapsulating profound wisdom on the strength of absolute devotion to his idol of worship-Ram.

Bhakti yoga is the be all and indeed, end all, of all forms of yoga. The word yoga has no meaning unless it is supported by bhakti, devotion, trust and complete surrender.

Krishna became a personal God for many and several groups across the world have become His staunch followers. They also created an institution of "Krishna Consciousness". But God cannot remain bound to a, or a select of groups, and by sheer definition has a universal presence (Omnipresent). Krishna was aware of this likely phenomenon, and he therefore placed Bhakti as the most important form of Yoga, available to everyone, regardless of any limitations.

He delivered the famous discourse of Bhagwat Gita in the middle of a war- Mahabharata, to Arjuna and took him through a journey of several forms of yoga, with an objective of making Arjuna realise his Dharma. Krishna was fully aware of the fact that Arjuna must realise his duties and responsibilities, not only towards his family and friends, but also in the larger interests of mankind to establish the rule of Dharma.

After exhibiting his Virat Swarup, whereupon Arjuna was left in no doubt about His true persona, Krishna resorts to the quintessential form of Bhakti yoga- complete surrender to only one power in the universe, which has no second. This embodies the supreme principle of Advaita-Vedanta (Non-duality). After educating Arjuna on all forms of yoga, each one according to Him has the potential of attaining enlightenment, Krishna suggests that Arjuna seek ultimate refuge in that one power- "Brahman" that alone is the embodiment of universal consciousness. Everything is an illusion and transient. He alone is existence-bliss-consciousness. (सत चित्त आनंद)

सर्वधर्मान्परित्यज्य मामेकं शरणं व्रज |
अहं त्वां सर्वपापेभ्यो मोक्षयिष्यामि मा शुचः || 66 || CH 18

sarva-dharmān parityajya mām ekaṁ śharaṇaṁ vraja
ahaṁ tvāṁ sarva-pāpebhyo mokṣhayiṣhyāmi mā śhuchaḥ

sarva-dharmān—all varieties of dharmas; parityajya—abandoning; mām—unto me; ekam—only; śharaṇam—take refuge; vraja—take; aham—I; tvām—you; sarva—all; pāpebhyaḥ—from sinful reactions; mokṣhayiṣhyāmi—shall liberate; mā—do not; śhuchaḥ—fear

Translation

Abandon all varieties of dharmas and simply surrender unto Me alone. I shall liberate you from all sinful reactions; do not fear.

Commentary

All along, Krishna had been asking Arjun to do two things simultaneously—engage his mind in devotion and engage his body in fulfilling his material duty as a warrior. He thus wanted Arjun not to give up his Kshatriya *dharma*, but to do devotion alongside with it. This is the principle of *karm yog*. Now, Krishna reverses this teaching by saying that here is no need to fulfil even material *dharma*. Arjun can renounce all material duties and simply surrender to God. This is the principle of *karm sanyās*. Here, one may question that if we give up all our material *dharmas* will we not incur sin? Krishna tells Arjun not to fear; he will absolve him from all sins and liberate him from material existence.

To comprehend this instruction of Krishna, we need to understand the term *dharma*. It comes from the root word *dhṛi*, which means *dhāraṇ karane yogya*, or "responsibilities, duties, thoughts, and actions that are appropriate for us." There are two kinds of *dharmas*—material *dharma* and spiritual *dharma*. These two kinds of *dharma* are based upon two different understandings of the "self." When we identify ourselves as the body, then our *dharma* is determined in accordance with our bodily designations, obligations, duties, and norms. Hence, serving the bodily parents, fulfilling the responsibilities to society, nation, etc. are all bodily *dharma*. This is also called *apara dharma* or material *dharma*. This includes the *dharma* as a Brahmin, Kshatriya, etc. However, when we identify ourselves as the soul, we have no material designations of *varṇa* (social class) and *āśhram* (status in life). The soul's Father, Mother, Friend, Beloved, and resting place are all God. Hence our one and only *dharma* becomes loving devotional service to God. This is also called *para dharma* or spiritual *dharma*.

If one leaves the material *dharma* it is considered a sin due to dereliction of duty. But if one leaves material *dharma* and takes the shelter of spiritual *dharma*, it is not a sin. The Śhrīmad Bhāgavatam states:

devarṣhi-bhūtāpta-nṛiṇāṁ pitṝīṇāṁ na kiṅkaro nāyam ṛiṇī cha rājan
sarvātmanā yaḥ śharaṇaṁ śharaṇyaṁ gato mukundaṁ parihṛitya kartam
(11.5.41) [v37]

This verse explains that for those who do not surrender to God, there are five debts—to the celestial gods, to the sages, to the ancestors, to other humans, and to other living beings. The *varṇāśhram* system includes various procedures for releasing ourselves from these five kinds of debts. However, when we surrender to God, we are automatically released from all these debts, just as by watering the roots of a tree, all its branches, twigs, leaves, flowers, and fruit automatically get watered. Similarly, by fulfilling our duty to God, we automatically fulfil our duty to everyone. Hence, there is no sin in renouncing material *dharma* if we are properly situated in spiritual *dharma*. In fact, the goal is to engage completely and wholeheartedly in spiritual *dharma*. The Shrīmad Bhāgavatam states:

ājñāyaivaṁ guṇān doṣhān mayādiṣhṭān api svakān
dharmān santyajya yaḥ sarvān māṁ bhajeta sa tu sattamaḥ (11.11.32)
[v38]

"I have given innumerable instructions regarding the performance of bodily *dharma* in the Vedas. But those who realize the shortcomings in these, and renounce all prescribed duties, to simply engage in my devotional service, I consider them to be the best *sādhaks*." In the Ramayana, we read how Lakshman renounced all material duties to accompany Lord Ram in the forest. He said:

guru pitu mātu na jānahu kāhū, kahahu subhāū nātha patiyāū
more sabahiñ eka tumha swāmī, dinabhandhu ura antarayamī [v39]

"O Lord, please believe me, I do not know any teacher, father, mother, etc. As far as I am concerned, you, the saviour of the fallen and the knower of the heart, are my Master and my everything." Similarly, Prahlad said:

mātā nāsti pitā na 'sti na 'sti me swajano janaḥ [v40]

"I do not know any mother, father, or relative (God is everything to me)." In the *Bhagavad Gita*, Krishna gave Arjun sequentially higher instructions. Initially, he instructed Arjun to do *karm*, i.e., his material *dharma* as a warrior (verse 2.31). But material *dharma* does not result in God-realization; it leads to the celestial abodes, and once the pious merits are depleted one must come back. Hence, Krishna next instructed Arjun to do *karm yog*, i.e., his material *dharma* with the body and spiritual *dharma* with the mind. He asked Arjun to fight the war with the body and remember God with the mind (verse 8.7). This instruction of *karm yog* forms the major portion of the Bhagavad Gita. Now in the very end, Shree Krishna instructs Arjun to practice *karm sanyās*, i.e., renounce all material *dharma* and simply adopt spiritual *dharma*, which is love for God. He should thus fight, not because it is his duty as a warrior, but because God wants him to do so.

Bhakti, devotion, surrender usually take two forms. It can be a silent chanting of the name or names of God, known as Jaap, or it can be in words spoken or sung in different languages. The significance of the 'word' in the context of Bhakti Yoga has been referred to in many faiths. For example, in Bible, King James version states that "In the beginning was the Word, and the Word was with God, and the Word was God". Every congregation in a church begins and ends with Hymns in the praise and glory of God.

In Vedanta, the Word ओम (OM) is regarded as the most primordial sound. Both science-in the Big Bang theory on the origin of the universe, and religious scriptures recognise ओम as the first sound. Further elaborating the importance of ओम, also referred to as प्रणव, Krishna in Chapter 8, verse 13 of Bhagwat Gita says.

ओमित्येकाक्षरं ब्रह्म व्याहरन्मामनुस्मरन् |
य: प्रयाति त्यजन्देहं स याति परमां गतिम् || 13 || CH 8

oṁ ityekākṣharaṁ brahma vyāharan mām anusmaran
yaḥ prayāti tyajan dehaṁ sa yāti paramāṁ gatim

One who departs from the body while remembering Me, the Supreme Personality, and chanting the syllable Om, will attain the supreme goal.

While singing hymns is the standard practice followed by Christians, Kirtan and singing of bhajans is the mainstay of Bhakti yoga performed by Hindus and faiths that have strong affinity with Vedanta. Sikhism for instance, believes in a continuous rendition of bhajans as Jaap from Guru Granth Sahib or Guru Bani. Meera bhai expressed her love and devotion for Krishna through Bhajans that have assumed an iconic form.

Whirling Dervishes of Turkey, an 800-year-old tradition that has been preserved on UNESCO's list of intangible Heritage of Humanity is quintessentially, Bhakti Yoga. A truly mesmerizing spectacle transports the viewers to the world of deep devotion.

Sufi music, its lyrics and music represent the highest form of Bhakti, where a devotee completely identifies himself with Allah and regards Him as his beloved. The concept of Bhakti is suffused with love, romance and surrender, not to the worldly relations, but for the one supernatural entity that is invisible, but presumed and believed to reside in everyone's heart.

One very profound feature of Bhakti Yoga is that all other forms of Yoga begin with Bhakti and eventually converge and indeed, merge into Bhakti Yoga. Performance of all Yoga and related practices, draw their sustenance from Bhakti and absolute faith, in the existence and power of that entity.

Bhakti yoga is unconditional and is characterised by complete surrender to the Almighty. There is no quid pro quo. A true devotee does not expect nor demands anything from the subject of his devotion. It is pure love that transcends everything material. Some of us make our devotion conditional upon receiving something from God, in exchange of the time and effort that we spend in worship or in visiting a temple or a place of pilgrimage. We negotiate with God and resolve that if we get what we want (Usually some material benefit), we will visit the holy shrine and make some offerings to please Him. There can be nothing more absurd than this. This is not Bhakti yoga. God sitting in his shrine, here or wherever we believe Him to be, is not distributing favours in exchange of a few moments of devotion or some material offerings. Everyone will get whatever he or she does, in accordance with his or her Karmas-that much and no more at the appropriate time, nor before or after. Deriding the tendency of Sankalp-resolution in exchange of the material benefits, Krishna in chapter 6 makes following assertions.

सङ्कल्पप्रभवान्कामांस्त्यक्त्वा सर्वानशेषत: |
मनसैवेन्द्रियग्रामं विनियम्य समन्तत: || 24 || CH 6

शनै: शनैरुपरमेद्बुद्ध्या धृतिगृहीतया |
आत्मसंस्थं मन: कृत्वा न किञ्चिदपि चिन्तयेत् || 25 || CH 6

sankalpa—a resolve; prabhavān—born of; kāmān—desires; tyaktvā—having abandoned; sarvān—all; aśheṣhataḥ—completely; manasā—through the mind; eva—certainly; indriya-grāmam—the group of senses; viniyamya—restraining; samantataḥ—from all sides; śhanaiḥ—gradually; śhanaiḥ—gradually; uparamet—attain peace; buddhyā—by intellect; dhṛiti-gṛihītayā—achieved through determination of resolve that is in accordance with scriptures; ātma-sanstham—fixed in God; manaḥ—mind; kritvā—having made; na—not; kiñchit—anything; api—even; chintayet—should think of

Translation

Completely renouncing all desires arising from thoughts of the world, one should restrain the senses from all sides with the mind. Slowly and steadily, with conviction in the intellect, the mind will become fixed in God alone, and will think of nothing else.

Commentary

Meditation requires the dual process of removing the mind from the world and fixing it on God. Here, Krishna begins by describing the first part of the process—taking the mind away from the world.

Thoughts of worldly things, people, events, etc. come to the mind when it is attached to the world. Initially, the thoughts are in the form of *sphurṇā* (flashes of feelings and ideas). When we insist on the implementation of *sphurṇā*, it becomes *saṅkalp*. Thus, thoughts lead to *saṅkalp* (pursuit of these objects) and *vikalp* (revulsion from them), depending upon whether the attachment is positive or negative. The seed of pursuit and revulsion grows into the plant of desire, "This should happen. This should not happen." Both *saṅkalp* and *vikalp* immediately create impressions on the mind, like the film of a camera exposed to the light. Thus, they directly impede meditation upon God. They also have a natural tendency to flare up, and a desire that is a seed today can become an inferno tomorrow. Thus, one who desires success in meditation should renounce the affinity for material objects.

Having described the first part of the process of meditation—removing the mind from the world—Krishna then talks of the second part. The mind should be made to reside upon God. He says this will not happen automatically, but with determined effort, success will come slowly.

Determination of resolve that is in accordance with the scriptures is called *dhṛiti*. This determination comes with conviction of the intellect. Many people acquire academic knowledge of the scriptures about the nature of the self and the futility of worldly pursuits. But their daily life is at variance with their knowledge, and they are seen to indulge in sin, sex, and intoxication. This happens because their intellect is not convinced about that knowledge. The power of discrimination comes with the conviction of the intellect about the impermanence of the world and the eternality of one's relationship with God. Thus, utilizing the intellect, one must gradually cease sensual indulgence. This is called *pratyāhār*, or control of the mind and senses from running toward the objects of the senses. Success in *pratyāhār* will not come immediately. It will be achieved through gradual and repeated exercise.

A true bhakta stays unruffled in moments of adversity and does not complain, does not cry and reposes his complete faith in the justice of the Almighty. In happiness and prosperity, he stays rooted in his belief and continues to worship with the same ardour as in grief. Kabir's profound words.

सुख की माथे सिल पड़े जो नाम हृदय से जाए
बलिहारी वा दुख के जो पल पल नाम जपाए

The concept of Bhakti is based on a deep personal connect with your chosen deity. Act of worship cannot be outsourced to any other individual. Some households with enough material resources but inadequate time, set up a small temple or a place of worship in one nice corner of their home. The place is duly sanctified, has statues of many gods and goddesses, including frills required to perform regular worship. Statues are carefully chosen and made of expensive marble or silver. Some members of the household regularly go inside the place of worship and as a routine, spend some time and feel good at the end of this visit. Regular pooja in some households (Where inmates are short on time and have resources) however, is performed by a pandit whose services are specially requisitioned for this purpose. In this situation, major share of the benefits of the worship, if at all will go to the pandit. Bhakti cannot be outsourced. Bhakti yoga really must go beyond the routine and cannot be reduced to an exercise performed out of compulsion.

Bhakti Yoga is open to everyone, especially if you are confronted with the issue of faith or lack of it. In the material context, most of us are driven by logic and rationality. We want proof for everything. The entire body of scientific development is based upon proof, empirical testing and validation. We use our sense organs, mind and intellect to arrive at proof. However, it is essential to understand that our natural endowments have their own limitations, and truth as we see it may be an illusion. Classic example of this is mirage in a desert. Driving through an expansive stretch of desert, a traveller completely dehydrated searches for water and sees an oasis at a distance. Reaching the spot, he sees nothing but more sand. This is true of all experiences given by our other sense organs. Reality may be different from what we see, hear or touch.

Inevitably, many of us then take recourse to the phenomenon of faith. Indeed, several scientists, hard core rationalists having reached the pinnacle of their glory in scientific domain were unable to explain several phenomena that take place in this vast universe. They eventually surrendered to the compelling mandates of faith. It must be said that faith is a very powerful instrument and is intrinsic to the human nature. In Gita, chapter 17, verses 2 & 3, Krishna categorically defines a human being as an embodiment of faith.

श्रीभगवानुवाच |
त्रिविधा भवति श्रद्धा देहिनां सा स्वभावजा |
सात्त्विकी राजसी चैव तामसी चेति तां शृणु || 2 || CH 17

śhrī-bhagavān uvācha
tri-vidhā bhavati śhraddhā dehināṁ sā svabhāva-jā
sāttvikī rājasī chaiva tāmasī cheti tāṁ śhṛiṇu

śhrī-bhagavān uvācha—the Supreme Personality said; tri-vidhā—of three kinds; bhavati—is; śhraddhā—faith; dehinām—embodied beings; sā—which; sva-bhāva-jā—born of one's innate nature; sāttvikī—of the mode of goodness; rājasī—of the mode of passion; cha—and; eva—certainly; tāmasī—of the mode of ignorance; cha—and; iti—thus; tām—about this; śhṛiṇu—hear

The Supreme Divine Personality said: Every human being is born with innate faith, which can be of three kinds—*sāttvic, rājasic,* or *tāmasic*. Now hear about this from Me.

Commentary

Nobody can be without faith, for it is an inseparable aspect of the human personality. Those who do not believe in the scriptures are also not bereft of faith. Their faith is reposed elsewhere. It could be on the logical ability of their intellect, or the perceptions of their senses, or the theories they have decided to believe in. For example, when people say, "I do not believe in God because I cannot see him," they do not have faith in God, but they have faith in their eyes. Hence, they assume that if their eyes cannot see something, it probably does not exist. This is also a kind of faith. Others say, "I do not believe in the authenticity of the ancient scriptures. Instead, I accept the theories of modern science." This is also a kind of faith, for we have seen in the last few centuries how theories of science keep getting amended and overthrown. It is possible that the present scientific theories we believe to be true may also be proved incorrect in the future. Accepting them as truths is also a leap of faith. Prof. Charles H. Townes, Nobel Prize winner in Physics, expressed this very nicely: "Science itself requires faith. We don't know if our logic is correct. I don't know if you are there. You don't know if I am here. We may just be imagining all this. I have a faith that the world is what it seems like, and thus I believe you are there. I can't prove it from any fundamental point of view… Yet I must accept a certain framework in which to operate. The idea that 'religion is faith' and 'science is knowledge,' I think, is quite wrong. We scientists believe in the existence of the external world and the validity of our own logic. We feel quite comfortable about it. Nevertheless, these are acts of faith. We can't prove them." Whether one is a material scientist, a social scientist, or a spiritual scientist, one cannot avoid the leap of faith required in the acceptance of knowledge.

Human beings are complete personification of faith. However, an immersive experience in Bhakti Yoga would occur when it is directed at a specific entity. That is the reason why a tradition of personal God became prevalent. Interestingly, while Vedanta Advaita recognises only one God-Brahman, Hindu Pantheon has deities who have evolved in countless numbers. It gives complete freedom to a devotee to worship God/gods/deity of one's own choice. Meera chose Krishna, Tulsidas worshipped Ram as his idol. There are Shiv-Bhakts, devotees of Lord Ganesh. In Eastern parts of India, Ma Durga/Kali is the main deity for the worshippers. They all are manifestations of one Brahman who appears in different forms, in different time-zones and diverse geographical areas. They exhibit distinct attributes and devotees choose one and worship Him or Her all their life. Lacs of temples have also spanned across the country. There is usually one presiding deity in one temple with a cohort of Gods, and devotees perform worship for the main God and do a subsidiary worship for others. The name of the temple gets it after the name of the presiding Deity.

*I*n many ways, the tradition of personal God helps the devotee in his devotional practice. It brings concentration and facilitates focus on one entity. This also helps him in Dhyana Yoga and surrender to one God becomes far easier than having to please many. Bhakti Yoga, unlike Raja Yoga is a non-stop connect with the chosen deity. The dominant emotion is love and this does not require any preparation, nor any special posture. In that sense, it is easy to adopt yet difficult to practise requiring the mandates of absolute surrender.

In certain quarters, there is a criticism of the practice of idol worship which indeed is the mainstay of classical Hinduism. This was primarily on account of exploitation of the impressionable masses by the Brahmanical order that became very powerful, arrogating to themselves the direct powers of God. They became the dispenser of mercy or the wrath of God 0n to the gullible individuals. This led to unrest and a rebellion by some members of the community who saw a nefarious design in the practice of religion in its pure form. Hinduism branched into other sects and religious groups such as Arya samaj movement, Sikhism that literally banned the practice of idol worship. Their ideologies, names of the deities, philosophy and the concept of the oneness of God remained unchanged. Only a few practices and rituals changed. For example, in Sikhism the service of mankind became the service of the God. In Arya samaj chanting of Vedic Mantras and practice of Yagna became prominent. Intermediaries such as Pandit and purohits were largely done away with.

However, in the Sanatana Dharma traditions, idol worship in temples with chanting of mantras, morning and evening aarti continued and in Hinduism, this continues to have the largest following. Many households performed the daily puja and rituals in a mini temple they set up in one nice room or a corner of their homes. There are clear reasons behind this tradition. Firstly, a temple became a preferred place for congregations on the occasions of religious festivals-these are far too many and there is always a tendency to celebrate it in a gathering, meeting people whom you may not see otherwise. Secondly, a temple, a place of worship is presumed to be sanctified by pure thoughts and chanting of mantras and bhajans by millions of people overtime. There is a perception and experience of peace and tranquillity within the precincts of such places. We all look for it even if it is short lived.

The most important reason, however, is to feel the personal presence of God in the form we humans are used to. All religions believe that God is immanent, present everywhere, all powerful, but that is part of our imagination. We are also told by the scriptures that God is Nirguna Nirakara-has no attributes, no image yet we want to see him in real physical form. God comes to the world in several incarnations (Avatars), and we make his image the way we see him. Hinduism has several avatars, and we have as many images and as many temples in the male/female forms.

God is everywhere, but its unmanifest presence becomes a challenge for the ordinary individual. He must see him in human shape and form. This is also essential for him to concentrate, perform Dhyana and seek spiritual realisation.

All of us need personal God (ईष्टदेव) to meditate upon and identify ourselves with.

This is exactly what Krishna says in the following verses.

क्लेशोऽधिकतरस्तेषामव्यक्तासक्तचेतसाम् ||
अव्यक्ता हि गतिर्दुःखं देहवद्भिरवाप्यते || 5 || CH 12

kleśho 'dhikataras teṣhām avyaktāsakta-chetasām
avyaktā hi gatir duḥkhaṁ dehavadbhir avāpyate

kleśhaḥ—tribulations; adhika-taraḥ—full of; teṣhām—of those; avyakta—to the unmanifest; āsakta—attached; chetasām—whose minds; avyaktā—the unmanifest; hi—indeed; gatiḥ—path; duḥkham—exceedingly difficult; deha-vadbhiḥ—for the embodied; avāpyate—is reached

Translation

For those whose minds are attached to the unmanifest, the path of realization is full of tribulations. Worship of the unmanifest is exceedingly difficult for embodied beings.

Commentary

Having embraced worshippers of all His various manifestations into the fold, Shree Krishna again reiterates His preference for the worship of the personal form. He surmises the worship of the impersonal Brahman by saying that it is an exceedingly challenging path that is full of tribulations.

Why is the worship of the formless Brahman so difficult? The first and foremost reason for this is that we humans possess a form ourselves and we have been habituated to interacting with forms in endless lifetimes. Thus, while striving to love God as well, if our mind has a wonderful, enchanting form to meditate upon, it can easily focus upon it and increase its attachment to the Lord. However, in the case of the formless, the intellect cannot conceive of it, and the mind and senses have no tangible object to relate to. So, both the endeavours of meditating on God and increasing the mind's attachment to Him become difficult.

Worship of Brahman is also difficult in comparison to that of *Bhagavān* for another reason. The difference in paths can be understood through the *markaṭ-kiśhore nyāya* (the logic of the baby) monkey, and *mārjār-kiśhore nyāya* (the logic of the baby kitten). The baby monkey is responsible for holding onto her mother's stomach; it is not helped by its mother. When the mother monkey jumps from one branch to another, the onus of clinging tightly onto the mother is upon the baby, and if it is unable to do so, it falls. In contrast, a kitten is very small and delicate, but the mother takes the responsibility of transporting it from one place to another, by holding the kitten from behind the neck and lifting it up. In the analogy, the devotees of the formless can be compared to the baby monkey and the devotees of the personal form can be compared to the baby kitten. Those who worship the formless Brahman have the onus of progressing on the path by themselves, because Brahman does not bestow grace upon them. Brahman is not only formless, but also without attributes.

It has been described as *nirguṇa* (without qualities), *nirviśheṣh* (without attributes), and *nirākār* (without form). From this, it follows that Brahman does not manifest the quality of grace. The *jñānīs* who worship God as *nirguṇa, nirviśheṣh,* and *nirākār*, have to rely entirely upon self-effort for progress. On the other hand, the personal form of God is an ocean of compassion and mercy. Hence, devotees of the personal form receive the help of divine support in their *sādhanā*. Based on the protection that God bestows upon His devotees, Shree Krishna stated in verse 9.31: "O son of Kunti, declare it boldly that no devotee of Mine is ever lost." *He confirms the same statement in the next two verses.*

ये तु सर्वाणि कर्माणि मयि संन्यस्य मत्पराः |
अनन्येनैव योगेन मां ध्यायन्त उपासते || 6 || CH 12

तेषामहं समुद्धर्ता मृत्युसंसारसागरात् |
भवामि नचिरात्पार्थ मय्यावेशितचेतसाम् || 7 || CH 12

ye tu sarvāṇi karmāṇi mayi sannyasya mat-parāḥ
ananyenaiva yogena māṁ dhyāyanta upāsate
teṣhām ahaṁ samuddhartā mṛityu-saṁsāra-sāgarāt
bhavāmi na chirāt pārtha mayy āveśhita-chetasām

ye—who; tu—but; sarvāṇi—all; karmāṇi—actions; mayi—to Me; sannyasya—dedicating; mat-parāḥ—regarding Me as the Supreme goal; ananyena—exclusively; eva—certainly; yogena—with devotion; mām—Me; dhyāyantaḥ—meditating; upāsate—worship; teṣhām—of those; aham—I; samuddhartā—the deliverer; mṛityu-saṁsāra-sāgarāt—from the ocean of birth and death; bhavāmi—(I) become; na—not; chirāt—after a long time; pārtha—Arjun, the son of Pritha; mayi—with Me; āveśhita chetasām—of those whose consciousness is united

Translation

But those who dedicate all their actions to Me, regarding Me as the Supreme goal, worshiping Me and meditating on Me with exclusive devotion, O Parth, I swiftly deliver them from the ocean of birth and death, for their consciousness is united with Me.

Commentary

Krishna reiterates that His devotees reach Him quickly. Firstly, with the personal form of God as the object of their devotion, they easily focus their mind and senses upon Him. They engage their tongue and ears in chanting and hearing the divine Names of God, their eyes in seeing the image of His divine form, their body in performing actions for His pleasure, their mind in thinking of His wonderful Pastimes and Virtues, and their intellect in contemplating upon His Glories. In this way, they quickly unite their consciousness with God.

Secondly, since such devotees continuously offer their hearts in uninterrupted bhakti, God quickly bestows His grace upon them and removes the obstacles on their path. For those who are in communion with Him, He dispels their ignorance with the lamp of knowledge. In this way, God Himself becomes the Savior of His devotees and delivers them from *mṛityu saṁsāra sāgarāt* (the cycle of life and death).

Bhakti yoga confers numerous benefits, both in the spiritual and the temporal domain. In the spiritual context, you stay connected with your God perpetually. You see Him in everything, and a continuous unbreakable connect with Him brings you closer to enlightenment, which indeed, is the goal of every individual.

In the worldly context, you offer everything to Him, all your thoughts and actions are an offering, a kind of devotion to Him and that gives you absolute peace and happiness. Again, everyone in the world seeks only that. In real terms, money and power is sought with an ultimate objective of acquiring peace, prosperity and happiness. In the words of Socrates "happiness is what all people desire: since it is always the end (goal) of our activities, it is an unconditional good". He adds further- "happiness does not depend on external things, but rather on how those things are used".

Bhakti Yoga does exactly that and creates, peace, happiness, indeed bliss not experienced in worldly or material things. It brings in a concept of absolute equality amongst all creation. Everyone is equal and there is no discrimination, thus eliminating any possibility of hatred or strife in the world.

Reading through the text of Bhagvad Gita, one can clearly discern Krishna' distinct partiality towards Bhakti Yoga over all other Yoga. This paradigm of Yoga has a universal approach and confers benefits immediately. This would be evident from the following verses of chapter 9.

अनन्याश्चिन्तयन्तो मां ये जनाः पर्युपासते |
तेषां नित्याभियुक्तानां योगक्षेमं वहाम्यहम् || 22 || CH 9

ananyāśh chintayanto māṁ ye janāḥ paryupāsate
teṣhāṁ nityābhiyuktānāṁ yoga-kṣhemaṁ vahāmyaham

ananyāḥ—always; chintayantaḥ—think of; mām—Me; ye—those who; janāḥ—persons; paryupāsate—worship exclusively; teṣhām—of them; nitya abhiyuktānām—who are always absorbed; yoga—supply spiritual assets; kṣhemam—protect spiritual assets; vahāmi—carry; aham—I

Translation

There are those who always think of Me and engage in exclusive devotion to Me. To them, whose minds are always absorbed in Me, I provide what they lack and preserve what they already possess.

Commentary

A mother never thinks of deserting her newborn helpless child who is entirely dependent upon her. The supreme and eternal mother of the soul is God. In this verse, God offers motherly assurance to souls who surrender exclusively to Him. The words used are *vahāmi aham,* meaning "I personally carry the burden of maintaining My devotees," just as a married man carries the burden of maintaining his wife and children. God promises two things. The first is yog—He bestows His devotees the spiritual assets they do not possess. The second is *kṣhem*—He protects the spiritual assets that His devotees already possess.

However, the condition He has placed for this is exclusive surrender. This can again be understood through the same analogy of the mother and child. A newborn baby is fully dependent upon its mother, who takes care of the baby's welfare entirely. The baby simply cries whenever it needs anything; the mother cleans it, feeds it, bathes it, etc. But when the baby becomes a five-year old child, it begins doing some actions for itself. To that extent the mother reduces her responsibilities. And when the same child becomes a youth and assumes all responsibilities, the mother relinquishes her responsibilities further. Now if the father comes home and asks, "Where is our son?" the mother replies, "He has not returned home after school. He must have gone for a movie with his friends." Her attitude is now more neutral toward him. But when the same boy was a five-year old, and had gotten delayed by ten minutes in returning home from school, both the mother and father would begin to worry and take an immediate action to trace him, and get him to the safety of home.

In this way, as the boy keeps assuming more responsibilities, his mother keeps relinquishing her responsibilities. God's law is the same. When we act from our independent will, thinking that we are the doers of our actions, and depend upon our own prowess and abilities, God does not bestow His grace. He merely notes our karmas and gives the result. When we surrender partially to Him and partially depend upon material crutches, God also partially bestows His grace upon us. And when we offer ourselves exclusively to Him, *māmekaṁ śharaṇaṁ vraja*, God bestows His complete grace and takes full responsibility, by preserving what we have and providing what we lack.

A logical corollary to this phenomenon can be described in the following words.

(If you do what you want to do, the result will be in the hands of God. If you do what God wants you to do, the result will be in your hands.)

Another very significant aspect of Bhakti is the concept of complete austerity. Devotion does not come with any cost, does not require any major investment. We may build temples, adorn God's idols with gold, silver or precious stones, offer Him the most expensive food, celebrate holy events with great pomp and show, but if it is not offered with love and devotion, it fails to please or propitiate Him. Indeed, He most willingly and happily accepts a modest offering of a leaf, fruit or plain water from His devotee who offers it with profound and abiding love. The following statement confirms this.

पत्रं पुष्पं फलं तोयं यो मे भक्त्या प्रयच्छति |
तदहं भक्त्युपहृतमश्नामि प्रयतात्मन: || 26 || CH 9

patraṁ puṣhpaṁ phalaṁ toyaṁ yo me bhaktyā prayachchhati
tadahaṁ bhaktyupahṛitam aśhnāmi prayatātmanaḥ

patram—a leaf; puṣhpam—a flower; phalam—a fruit; toyam—water; yaḥ—who; me—to Me; bhaktyā—with devotion; prayachchhati—offers; tat—that; aham—I; bhakti-upahṛitam—offered with devotion; aśhnāmi—partake; prayata-ātmanaḥ—one in pure consciousness

Translation

If one offers to Me with devotion a leaf, a flower, some fruit, or even water, I delightfully partake of that item offered with love by My devotee in pure consciousness.

Commentary

Having established the benefits of worshipping the Supreme, Krishna now explains how easy it is to do so. In the worship of the *devatās* and the ancestors, there are many rules to propitiate them, which must be strictly followed. But God accepts anything that is offered with a loving heart. If you have some fruits, offer it to God, and He will be pleased. If there is no fruit available, offer Him a flower. If it is not the season for flowers, offer God a mere leaf; even that will suffice, provided it is a gift of love. If leaves are also scarce, make an offering of water, which is available everywhere, but ensure again that you do it with devotion. The word *bhaktyā* has been used in both the first and second lines of the verse. It is the bhakti of the devotee that is pleasing to God, and not the worth of the offering.

By making this wonderful statement, Krishna reveals the merciful divine nature of God. He is not concerned with the material value of our offering. Rather, He values, above everything else, the love with which we make the offering. Thus, the Hari Bhakti Vilas states:

tulasī-dala-mātreṇa jalasya chulukena cha
vikrīṇīte svam ātmānaṁ bhaktebhyo bhakta-vatsalaḥ (11.261)

"If you offer God with sincere love, just a *Tulsī* leaf and as much water as you can hold in your palm, He will offer Himself to you in return because He is endeared by love." How wonderful it is that the Supreme Master of unlimited universes, whose glorious qualities and virtues are amazing beyond description, and by whose mere thought multitudes of universes come into existence and disappear again, accepts even the humblest offering of His devotee that is given with genuine love. The word used here is *prayatātmanaḥ*, implying, "I accept the offerings of those whose hearts are pure."

The Shreemad Bhagavatam contains the same verse as the above verse of the Bhagavad Gita. While eating dry rice at the house of His friend, Sudama, Shree Krishna said:

patraṁ puṣhpaṁ phalaṁ toyaṁ yo me bhaktyā prayachchhati
tadahaṁ bhaktyupahṛitam aśhnāmi prayatātmanaḥ (10.81.4)

"If one offers Me with devotion, a leaf, a flower, a fruit, or even water, I delightfully partake of that article offered with love by My devotee in pure consciousness."

Whenever God descends upon the earth, He exhibits this quality in His divine Pastimes. Before the Mahabharat war, when Krishna went to Hastinapur to explore the possibility of fashioning an agreement between the Kauravas and Pandavas, the evil Duryodhan proudly prepared for Him a meal with fifty-six different items, (**56 भोग**). However, Krishna refused his hospitality and instead went to the humble hut of Vidurani, who had been longing deeply for the opportunity to serve her beloved Lord. Vidurani was overjoyed on receiving the Supreme Lord at her home. All she had to offer was bananas, but her mind was so benumbed with loving sentiments that she did not even realize she was dropping the fruit and putting the banana peels in His mouth. Nevertheless, seeing her devotion, Krishna blissfully ate the peels, as if they were the most delicious food in the world.

We all recognize and accept God as the creator of the universe. He surely is its owner too. All that we have in the material world is owned and provided by Him. The proportion of what is available to each one of us may vary in accordance with our effort and Karmas. His resources are inexhaustible and no one in the world, not even one individual can match the wealth and resources owned by Him. Any amount of material wealth, therefore, is not enough to please Him. How much can we give to the owner and the giver of all. Offerings in Bhakti are completely antithetical to materiality.

He needs pure love, devotion and surrender. These are the finest offerings to Him. A true Bhakt understands it abstains from ostentatious offerings.

यत्करोषि यदश्नासि यज्जुहोषि ददासि यत् |
यत्तपस्यसि कौन्तेय तत्कुरुष्व मदर्पणम् || 27 ||

yat karoṣhi yad aśhnāsi yaj juhoṣhi dadāsi yat
yat tapasyasi kaunteya tat kuruṣhva mad-arpaṇam

yat—whatever; karoṣhi—you do; yat—whatever; aśhnāsi—you eat; yat—whatever; juhoṣhi—offer to the sacred fire; dadāsi—bestow as a gift; yat—whatever; yat—whatever; tapasyasi—austerities you perform; kaunteya—Arjun, the son of Kunti; tat—them; kuruṣhva—do; mad arpaṇam—as an offering to Me

Translation

Whatever you do, whatever you eat, whatever you offer as oblation to the sacred fire, whatever you bestow as a gift, and whatever austerities you perform, O son of Kunti, do them as an offering to Me.

Commentary

In the previous verse, Krishna stated that all objects should be offered to Him. Now He says that all actions should also be offered to Him. Whatever social duties one may be engaged in, whatever food one may be eating, whatever beverages one may be drinking, whatever Vedic rites one may perform, whatever vows and austerities one may observe, should all be offered mentally to the Supreme Lord. Very often, people separate devotion from their daily life, and look on it as something that is only to be performed inside the temple room. However, devotion is not to be restricted to the periphery of the temple room; it is to be engaged in at every moment of our life.

Sage Narad defines bhakti in this manner:

nāradastu tadarpitā khilāchāratā tadvismaraṇe paramavyākulateti
(Nārad Bhakti Darśhan, *Sūtra* 19)

"Devotion means offering your every activity to God, and feeling intense separation if ever you lose remembrance of Him." When works are dedicated and mentally delivered to God, it is called *arpaṇam*. Such an attitude metamorphoses the mundane activities of material life into divine service of God. Swami Vivekananda expressed this attitude toward work when he declared: "No work is secular. Everything is devotion and service." Saint Kabir stated this in his couplet:

jahañ jahañ chalūñ karūñ parikramā, jo jo karūñ so sevā
jaba sovūñ karūñ daṇḍavat, jānūñ deva na dūjā

"Wherever I walk, I feel I am circumambulating the Lord's temple; whatever I do, I see it as service to God. When I go to sleep, I meditate on the sentiment that I am offering obeisance to God. In this way, I remain ever united with Him." Without realizing its significance, many people say the following verse in temples:

kāyena vāchā manasendriyair vā buddhyātmanā vānusṛita-svabhāvāt
karoti yad yat sakalaṁ parasmai nārāyaṇāyeti samarpayet tat
(Bhagavatam 11.2.36)

"Whatever one does with body, words, mind, senses, and intellect, in accordance with one's individual nature, should be offered to the Supreme Lord Narayan." However, this act of offering is not to be done at the end of the work by merely reciting mantras, such as *śhrī kṛiṣhṇāya samarpaṇam astu*, etc., as is done in the Vedic rituals. It is to be done while performing the action itself, by maintaining the consciousness that we are working for the pleasure of the Lord. *Having stated that all works should be offered to Him, Shree Krishna now lists the benefits of doing so.*

**शुभाशुभफलैरेवं मोक्ष्यसे कर्मबन्धनैः ।
संन्यासयोगयुक्तात्मा विमुक्तो मामुपैष्यसि ॥ 28 ॥ CH 9**

*śhubhāśhubha-phalair evaṁ mokṣhyase karma-bandhanaiḥ
sannyāsa-yoga-yuktātmā vimukto mām upaiṣhyasi*

śhubha aśhubha phalaiḥ—from good and bad results; evam—thus; mokṣhyase—you shall be freed; karma—work; bandhanaiḥ—from the bondage; sanyāsa-yoga—renunciation of selfishness; yukta-ātmā—having the mind attached to Me; vimuktaḥ—liberated; mām—to Me; upaiṣhyasi—you shall reach

Translation

By dedicating all your works to Me, you will be freed from the bondage of good and bad results. With your mind attached to Me through renunciation, you will be liberated and will reach Me.

Commentary

Every action has defects, just as fire is covered by smoke. When we walk on the earth, we unknowingly kill millions of tiny living entities. In our occupational duties, no matter how careful we are in the fulfilment of our duties, we still end up harming the environment and hurting others. Even if we eat a cup of yogurt, we still incur the sin of destroying the living entities that reside in it. Some religious sects try to reduce this involuntary killing by tying a cloth over their mouth. Even this does not fully eliminate the destruction of living entities in our breath.

When we perform our actions with the intention of fulfilling our self-interest, we are culpable for the sins we commit, knowingly or unknowingly. In accordance with the law of karma, we must reap their karmic reactions. Good works can also be binding because they oblige the soul to go to the celestial abodes to enjoy their results. Thus, both bad and good karmas result in the continuity of the cycle of birth and death. However, in this verse, Krishna gives a simple solution for destroying all karmic reactions of work. He uses the word *sanyās yog*, meaning renunciation of selfishness. He says that when we dedicate our actions for the pleasure of the Lord, we are freed from the fetters of both good and bad results.

Those who establish themselves in such consciousness are called *yog yuktātmā* (united in consciousness with God). Such yogis become *jīvan mukt* (liberated in consciousness) even in this body. And, upon leaving their mortal frame, they receive a divine body and eternal service in the divine Abode of God.

समोऽहं सर्वभूतेषु न मे द्वेष्योऽस्ति न प्रियः |
ये भजन्ति तु मां भक्त्या मयि ते तेषु चाप्यहम् || 29 || CH 9

samo 'haṁ sarva-bhūteṣhu na me dveṣhyo 'sti na priyaḥ
ye bhajanti tu māṁ bhaktyā mayi te teṣhu chāpyaham

samaḥ—equally disposed; aham—I; sarva-bhūteṣhu—to all living beings; na—no one; me—to Me; dveṣhyaḥ—inimical; asti—is; na—not; priyaḥ—dear; ye—who; bhajanti—worship with love; tu—but; mām—Me; bhaktyā—with devotion; mayi—reside in Me; te—such persons; teṣhu—in them; cha—and; api—also; aham—I

Translation

I am equally disposed to all living beings; I am neither inimical nor partial to anyone. But the devotees who worship Me with love reside in Me and I reside in them.

Commentary

We all intuitively believe that if there is a God, He must be perfectly just; there cannot be an unjust God. People suffering injustice in the world make statements such as, "Mr. Billionaire, you have the power of money on your side. Do what you like. God will settle our dispute. He is watching and will punish you. You cannot escape." This sort of statement does not indicate that the person making it is a saint, possessing absolute faith in God, for even common persons believe that God is perfectly just.

However, the previous verse by Krishna creates the doubt that God is partial toward His devotees, because while everyone is subject to the law of karma, God releases His devotees from it. Isn't this symptomatic of the defect of partiality? Krishna feels it necessary to clarify this point and begins the verse by saying *samo' ham,* meaning, "No, no, I am equal to all. But I have a uniform law in accordance with which I bestow My grace." This law was previously stated in verse 4.11: "In whatever way people surrender unto Me, I reciprocate accordingly. Everyone follows my path, knowingly or unknowingly, O son of Pritha."

ये यथा मां प्रपद्यन्ते तांस्तथैव भजाम्यहम् |
मम वर्त्मानुवर्तन्ते मनुष्या: पार्थ सर्वश: || 11 || CH 4

ye yathā māṁ prapadyante tāns tathaiva bhajāmyaham
mama vartmānuvartante manuṣhyāḥ pārtha sarvaśhaḥ

ye—who; yathā—in whatever way; mām—unto me; prapadyante—surrender; tān—them; tathā—so; eva—certainly; bhajāmi—reciprocate; aham—I; mama—my; vartma—path; anuvartante—follow; manuṣhyāḥ—men; pārtha—Arjun, the son of Pritha; sarvaśhaḥ—in all respects

Translation

In whatever way people surrender unto Me, I reciprocate accordingly. Everyone follows My path, knowingly or unknowingly, O son of Pritha.

Commentary

Here Krishna states that he reciprocates with everyone as they surrender to him. For those who deny the existence of God, he meets them in the form of the law of karma—he sits inside their hearts, notes their actions, and dispenses the results. But such atheists too cannot get away from serving him; they are obliged to serve God's material energy, Maya, in its various apparitions, as wealth, luxuries, relatives, prestige, etc. Maya holds them under the sway of anger, lust, and greed. On the other hand, for those who turn their mind away from worldly attractions and look upon God as the goal and refuge, he takes care of them just as a mother takes care of her child.

Krishna uses the word *bhajāmi*, which means "to serve." He serves the surrendered souls, by destroying their accumulated karmas of endless lifetimes, cutting the bonds of Maya, removing the darkness of material existence, and bestowing divine bliss, divine knowledge, and divine love. And when the devotee learns to love God selflessly, he willingly enslaves himself to their love. Shree Ram thus tells Hanuman:

ekaikasyopakārasya prāṇān dāsyāmi te kape
śheṣhasyehopakārāṇāṁ bhavām ṛiṇino vayaṁ
(Vālmīki Ramayan)[v14]

"O Hanuman, to release myself from the debt of one service you performed for me, I shall have to offer my life to you.

For all the other devotional services done by you, I shall remain eternally indebted." In this way, God reciprocates with everyone as they surrender to him.

Bhakti has that power where even God is obliged to surrender to His Bhakt in exchange of his devotion. What a simple and a beautiful way of creating a debt on God. A true devotee keeps accumulating this debt merely by worshiping Him and seeks discharge of this debt when he needs it. However, if you keep piling this debt on God without encashing it you get enlightenment before long. Ask nothing in return except His grace and devotion, and you will be bestowed with love and bliss.

Narendra before he became to be known as Vivekananda belonged to a middle-class family of Kolkata. His father the main earning member of the family died early, and the family were stuck in poverty. His brother was also not earning anything, and they had problems of managing even a square meal. In utter despair, Vivekananda went to Swami Ramkrishna and told him about this and pleaded with him to do something about it. Vivekananda requested Ramakrishna to ask Ma Kali to help the family with some basic provisions. Ramakrishna told Vivekananda that why don't you go and seek Her benevolence. Vivekananda hesitated and said that you are Her devotee, and She would listen to you. Ramakrishna insisted that he goes and ask for whatever he needs, himself. Vivekananda went to Kali temple and after a while came back. Ramakrishna asked him whether he got what he wanted. Vivekananda replied that when he went to the temple, he forgot to ask anything material. He only asked for Her grace, worship and blessings. Ramakrishna sent him back again and Vivekananda came back with the same answer. This happened two-three time with the same result. When asked by Ramakrishna, he replied when I reached there the only thought that came to my mind was to seek her blessings The story is that when Vivekananda reached home that night, there were plenty of provisions and food for the family. God has His own way of providing for His devotees. You don't need to ask anything but His grace.

The rainwater falls equally upon the earth. Yet, the drop that falls on the cornfields gets converted into grain; the drop that falls on the desert bush gets converted into a thorn; the drop that falls in the gutter becomes dirty water; and the drop that falls in the oyster becomes a pearl. There is no partiality on the part of the rain, since it is equitable in bestowing its grace upon the land. The raindrops cannot be held responsible for this variation in results, which are a consequence of the nature of the recipient. Similarly, God states here that He is equally disposed toward all living beings, and yet, those who do not love

Him are bereft of the benefits of His grace because their hearts are unsuitable vessels for receiving it. *So, what can people do whose hearts are impure? Krishna now reveals the purifying power of bhakti.*

क्षिप्रं भवति धर्मात्मा शश्वच्छान्तिं निगच्छति |
कौन्तेय प्रतिजानीहि न मे भक्त: प्रणश्यति || 31 || CH 9

kṣhipraṁ bhavati dharmātmā śhaśhvach-chhāntiṁ nigachchhati
kaunteya pratijānīhi na me bhaktaḥ praṇaśhyati

kṣhipram—quickly; bhavati—become; dharma-ātmā—virtuous; śhaśhvat-śhāntim—lasting peace; nigachchhati—attain; kaunteya—Arjun, the son of Kunti; pratijānīhi—declare; na—never; me—My; bhaktaḥ—devotee; praṇaśhyati—perishes

Translation

Quickly they become virtuous and attain lasting peace. O son of Kunti, declare it boldly that no devotee of Mine is ever lost.

Commentary

How can devotees be considered venerable, merely for having made the correct resolve? Krishna explains that if they continue the process of exclusive devotion with unflinching faith in God, their hearts will become purified, and they will swiftly develop saintly virtues.

Divine virtues emanate from God Himself. He is perfectly just, truthful, compassionate, loving, merciful, etc. Since we souls are His tiny parts, we are all naturally drawn to these godly qualities. But the process of becoming virtuous remains an elusive mystery. From childhood, we have heard that we must speak the truth, serve others, be free from anger, etc. and yet we are unable to put those teachings into practice for the simple reason that our mind is impure. Without purification of the mind, blemishes of character cannot be eradicated fully and permanently.

satya ahinsā ādi mana! bina hari bhajana na pāya
jala te ghṛita nikale nahīñ, koṭina kariya upāya (Bhakti Śhatak verse 35)

"Oil stains on a cloth cannot be removed by water, no matter how much we try. Similarly, truthfulness, non-violence, and other virtuous qualities cannot be acquired without engaging in devotion to God." These qualities manifest when the mind is purified; and the purification of the mind cannot take place without attaching it to the all-pure God.

Further, Krishna asks Arjun to boldly declare that His devotees will never perish. He does not say, "The *jñānī* (person of knowledge) will not be lost." Nor does He say, "The *karmī* (performer of rituals) shall not perish." He makes His promise for His *bhaktas* (devotees), saying that "they shall never come to ruin." Thereby, He reiterates what He had stated in verse 9.22, that He personally carries the burden of maintaining those who depend upon Him and engage in exclusive devotion unto Him.

It may seem intriguing why Krishna asks Arjun to make this statement, instead of declaring it Himself? The reason is that under special circumstances the Lord sometimes breaks His word, but He never permits His devotees' word to be broken. For example, Krishna had resolved that He would not lift weapons during the Mahabharat war. But when Bheeshma, considered the perfect devotee, resolved that he would either kill Arjun by sunset the next day or make the Lord lift weapons to protect him, Krishna broke His own vow to protect the vow made by Bheeshma. Thus, to reaffirm the strength of His statement, Krishna here says, "Arjun, you declare that My devotee will never perish, for I shall guarantee that your word will be kept."

मन्मना भव मद्भक्तो मद्याजी मां नमस्कुरु |
मामेवैष्यसि युक्त्वैवमात्मानं मत्परायण: || 34 || CH 9

man-manā bhava mad-bhakto mad-yājī māṁ namaskuru
mām evaiṣhyasi yuktvaivam ātmānaṁ mat-parāyaṇaḥ

mat-manāḥ—always think of Me; bhava—be; mat—My; bhaktaḥ—devotee; mat—My; yājī—worshipper; mām—to Me; namaskuru—offer obeisances; mām—to Me; eva—certainly; eṣhyasi—you will come; yuktvā—united with Me; evam—thus; ātmānam—your mind and body; mat-parāyaṇaḥ—having dedicated to Me

Translation

Always think of Me, be devoted to Me, worship Me, and offer obeisance to Me. Having dedicated your mind and body to Me, you will certainly come to Me.

Commentary

Having stressed bhakti, the path of devotion, throughout this chapter, Krishna now concludes it by entreating Arjun to become His devotee. He asks Arjun to unite his consciousness with God in true Yog, by worshipping Him, engaging the mind in meditation upon His divine form, and offering obeisance in pure humility to Him.

Namaskuru (the act of humble obeisance) effectively neutralizes vestiges of egotism that may arise in the performance of devotion. Thus, free from pride, with the heart immersed in devotion, one should dedicate all one's thoughts and actions to the Supreme. Krishna assures Arjun that such complete communion with Him through *bhakti-yoga* will result in the attainment of God-realization; of this, there should be no doubt.

Worship of God and Bhakti yoga is a kind of an investment we make through the medium of his worship. Every time we speak His name, remember Him with no other distraction, with our heart and mind fully immersed in Him, we enhance our spiritual wealth. We stay on this path and our wealth increases in proportion to the time we spent worshipping Him. We invest money in many instruments with a desire to have more of it, spend it, enjoy the benefits of larger wealth, get greater happiness and pleasure and feel secure.

A comparison between the two forms of investments will reveal huge differences in terms of the benefits that will come your way. Eventual goals of both these forms are happiness, peace and security. Money, more money and power that money usually brings in the material world has never fully assured the achievement of the goals mentioned above. Spiritual wealth will ensure it and ensure it on a long-term sustainable basis. Worldly wealth will diminish, sometime at a much faster pace, used up, damaged, stolen and lead to arrogance-a sure sign of decline. Spiritual wealth never diminishes. It gets bigger, stronger and ensures perennial peace and bliss. Return on Investment (ROI) in spiritual instruments far exceeds the one in the material world. Interestingly, it does not go away, birth after births and can be encashed at will. It will be interesting to look at the lyrics of a famous Meera Bhajan.

खर्च ना खूटे चोर ना लूटे खर्च ना खूटे चोर ना लूटे
दिन दिन बढ़त सवायो
पायो जी मैंने दिन दिन बढ़त सवायो
पायो जी मैंने राम रतन धन पायो पायो जी मैंने राम रतन धन पायो

Every word spoken in remembering Him creates a debt on Him. This debt does not require any monetary investment from us. Krishna says in Gita that I readily accept leaves, fruits or flowers offered to me by my devotee with love and faith. All material possessions are left behind in this world and no matter how much you earned in your lifetime on earth, it gets relinquished at once. You cannot claim it ever, including any debt you may have given to someone here. But the debt you create on God by worshipping Him stays with you for ever, here and hereinafter. He undertakes to protect it and deliver to you when you need it. That is the concept of Yogkhshem (योग क्षेम) Gita-CH 9/22

Bhakti Yoga may appear simple because it apparently does not require any overt action. Yet it demands complete surrender even while being engaged in regular activities that are essential. Swami Ramakrishna Paramhans used to say that God has given us two hands, Keep doing your work with one hand and worship God with the other. Once work is over, join the other hand as well in the worship of the Almighty.

Bhakti symbolises the highest form of spirituality which helps us transcend the ego which constitutes the biggest impediment in our journey of self-realisation. Unconditional love which is the hallmark of Bhakti yoga is the strongest antidote to ego. An exaggerated opinion of the self leads to arrogance and is a sure recipe for decline and conflicts in interpersonal relationships. Intellectual arrogance with a boost of ego spells disaster for all concerned. History is replete with examples of people achieving greatness in several disciplines such as politics, science, religion, but their arrogance has been their undoing. Acquisition of unlimited power and knowledge, unsupported by devotion has led some to become megalomaniac and start playing God. This alone in time has proved to be their nemesis.

There is a story of an interesting conversation between two friends-a scientist and a philosopher. The scientist had spent major part of his life in research in biology and life-sciences. He was a non-believer but a great scientist. The two met and the scientist told the philosopher friend that he does not believe in God and indeed, he does not believe in His existence. His research and experiment have shown him that he can produce life in a laboratory without any external help. So, the two friends went to his LAB and the scientist started his preparations for creating life. He then asked his philosopher friend to get some part of the earth. His immediate response was “get your own piece of earth. The one that you are asking for belongs to God”.

Ownership of whatever is present in the universe must vest with the creator. Our world is self-sufficient and everything that exists here belongs to Him. All animate and inanimate entities are created here and here only they dissolve. We work under several illusions and one of these relates to a statement we often make about our entrance and exit from the world. We mention that we come into this world at birth and go out of the world at death. Human body, or for that matter every living being is made of five elements (पंचभूत). These are- Earth, water, air, fire and sky. All these five elements are present right here and are not imported from any other part of the universe. Nature uses a biological process to put these five elements together and a life is created. These five elements interact and impact our bodies, and in due course of time, the body declines and perishes. The decomposition of the gross body results in the same amount of five elements going back to world whence it got created. We don't come into this world, nor we go out of this world. This way God is never short on the availability of the raw material to go on the task of creation.

There is one entity that uses our body as a temporary abode, and leaves when the body perishes. We have given it several names-Atma, Soul, Consciousness, Awareness. That indeed is our identity.

The correct statement would be, "We come out of this world, and we go back into the world".

Bhakti is the platform and a scaffold on which all other forms of Yogas rest. You may pursue or engage in any form of Yoga practice but if the component of Bhakti is missing, it ceases to create any value or has little or no significance.

CHAPTER THREEE

KARMA YOGA

Yoga in everyone's life.

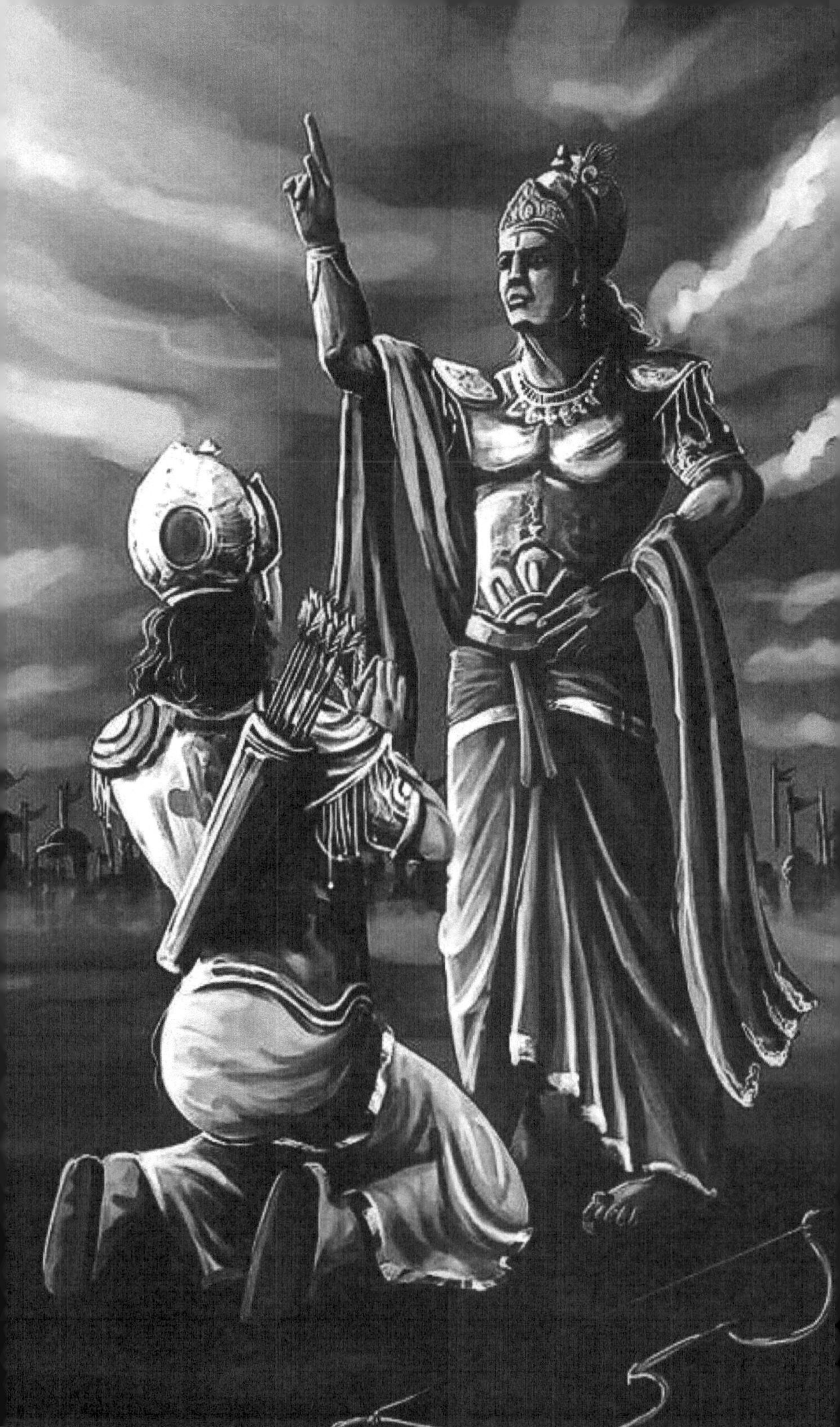

KARAMYOGA

The etymological origin of the word Karma is traced to the Sanskrit 'Kri', to do; all actions are Karma. A wider definition of Karma would include the effects of actions as well. Performance of Karma is mandatory for all human beings. Verse 3 chapters 5 of Bhagwat Gita makes a categorical statement in this regard.

न हि कश्चित्क्षणमपि जातु तिष्ठत्यकर्मकृत् |
कार्यते ह्यवश: कर्म सर्व: प्रकृतिजैर्गुणै: || 5 || CH 3

na hi kaśhchit kṣhaṇam api jātu tiṣhṭhatyakarma-kṛit
kāryate hyavaśhaḥ karma sarvaḥ prakṛiti-jair guṇaiḥ

na—not; hi—certainly; kaśhchit—anyone; kṣhaṇam—a moment; api—even; jātu—ever; tiṣhṭhati—can remain; akarma-kṛit—without action; kāryate—are performed; hi—certainly; avaśhaḥ—helpless; karma—work; sarvaḥ—all; prakṛiti-jaiḥ—born of material nature; guṇaiḥ—by the qualities

Translation

There is no one who can remain without action even for a moment. Indeed, all beings are compelled to act by their qualities born of material nature (the three *guṇas*).

Commentary

Some people think that action refers only to professional work, and not to daily activities such as eating, drinking, sleeping, waking and thinking. So, when they renounce their profession, they think they are not performing actions. But Krishna considers all activities performed with the body, mind, and tongue as actions. Hence, he tells Arjun that complete inactivity is impossible even for a moment. If we simply sit down, it is an activity; if we lie down, that is also an activity; if we fall asleep, the mind is still engaged in dreaming; even in deep sleep, the heart and other bodily organs are functioning. Thus, Krishna declares that for human beings' complete inactivity is an impossible state, since the body-mind-intellect mechanism is compelled by its own construct of the three *guṇas* (*sattva, rajas,* and *tamas*) to perform work in the world. The Śhrīmad Bhāgavatam contains a similar verse:

na hi kaśhchit kṣhaṇam api jātu tiṣhṭhaty akarma-kṛit
kāryate hy avaśhaḥ karma guṇaiḥ svābhāvikair balāt (6.1.53) [v1]

"Nobody can remain inactive for even a moment. Everyone is forced to act by their modes of nature."

There is no one who can remain without work even for a moment. Our material nature influenced by three gunas, (satvik, rajasik, tamsik) force us to perform and act incessantly. Karma broadly, comprises thought, speech and action. Karma is not limited to the normal activities that everyone ordinarily performs, such as eating, drinking, sleeping, walking, talking etc. It has much wider connotations. In our state of sleep, we breathe, our heart beats both voluntarily and involuntarily, we stay in a state of action. Our body-mind-intellect combination is perpetually working, overtly or covertly.

नियतं कुरु कर्म त्वं कर्म ज्यायो ह्यकर्मण: |
शरीरयात्रापि च ते न प्रसिद्ध्येदकर्मण: || ८ ||

niyataṁ kuru karma tvaṁ karma jyāyo hyakarmaṇaḥ
śharīra-yātrāpi cha te na prasiddhyed akarmaṇaḥ

niyatam—constantly; kuru—perform; karma—Vedic duties; tvam—you; karma—action; jyāyaḥ—superior; hi—certainly; akarmaṇaḥ—than inaction; śharīra—bodily; yātrā—maintenance; api—even; cha—and; te—your; na prasiddhyet—would not be possible; akarmaṇaḥ—inaction

Translation

You should thus perform your prescribed Vedic duties, since action is superior to inaction. By ceasing activity, even your bodily maintenance will not be possible.

Commentary

Until the mind and intellect reach a state where they are absorbed in God-consciousness, physical work performed in an attitude of duty is very beneficial for one's internal purification. Hence, the Vedas prescribe duties for humans, to help them discipline their mind and senses. In fact, laziness is described as one of the biggest pitfalls on the spiritual path:

ālasya hi manuṣhyāṇāṁ śharīrastho mahān ripuḥ
nāstyudyamasamo bandhūḥ kṛitvā yaṁ nāvasīdati [v4]

"Laziness is the greatest enemy of humans and is especially pernicious since it resides in their own body. Work is their most trustworthy friend and is a guarantee against downfall." Even the basic bodily activities like eating, bathing, and maintaining proper health require work. These obligatory actions are called *nitya karm*. To neglect these basic maintenance activities is not a sign of progress, but an indication of slothfulness, leading to emaciation and weakness of both body and mind. On the other hand, a cared for and nourished body is a positive adjunct on the road to spirituality. Thus, the state of inertia does not lend itself either to material or spiritual achievement. For the progress of our own soul, we should embrace the duties that help elevate and purify our mind and intellect.

Further elaborating on the necessity of work, Krishna says that you need to perform your prescribed duty as action, because action is superior to inaction. Even maintenance of the body or survival is not possible in the state of inaction. The next question that logically follows is regarding the kind of Karma-what, when how and why. The answer to the 'why' has been appropriately answered in the previous paragraphs. We need now to address other related questions.

The primary mover of all our actions rests in our intellect/mind where all thoughts are born. We must make a distinction between some actions that we perform daily, and these assume a familiar pattern and become routine tasks-eating drinking walking sleeping, and after a while these are done in an automation mode. Largely, we do these actions in a state of unawareness, and this becomes a mechanical exercise.

Recognizing the importance and primacy of thought, Maitri Upanishad, drawn from Vedanta says.

"One's thought is one's world. What a person thinks, is what he becomes".
In the context of Karam Yoga, our thoughts assume great significance. Indeed, our speech and actions are driven by our thoughts and hence they must be subservient to our thoughts, follow them and not precede them. Any word spoken or any action performed without thoughts, has the potential of getting us in trouble. It may also cause irreparable collateral damage to our relationships, work and spoil our reputation.

While Bhagwat Gita covers a wide spectrum of our existence and is rightly described as 'a way of life' by many philosophers, thought leaders, religious personalities and scholars of Indian scriptures, the chief element that everyone associates with it, relates to Karama yoga. One verse that is on the lips of everyone who has some knowledge of Gita is verse 47, chapter 2.

कर्मण्येवाधिकारस्ते मा फलेषु कदाचन |
मा कर्मफलहेतुर्भूर्मा ते सङ्गोऽस्त्वकर्मणि || 47 || CH 2

karmaṇy-evādhikāras te mā phaleṣhu kadāchana
mā karma-phala-hetur bhūr mā te saṅgo 'stvakarmaṇi

karmaṇi—in prescribed duties; eva—only; adhikāraḥ—right; te—your; mā—not; phaleṣhu—in the fruits; kadāchana—at any time; mā—never; karma-phala—results of the activities; hetuḥ—cause; bhūḥ—be; mā—not; te—your; saṅgaḥ—attachment; astu—must be; akarmaṇi—in inaction

Translation

You have a right to perform your prescribed duties, but you are not entitled to the fruits of your actions. Never consider yourself to be the cause of the results of your activities, nor be attached to inaction.

Commentary

This is an extremely popular verse of the *Bhagavat Gita*, so much so that even most school children in India are familiar with it. It offers deep insight into the proper spirit of work and is often quoted whenever the topic of *karm yog* is discussed. The verse gives four instructions regarding the science of work: 1) Do your duty, but do not concern yourself with the results. 2) The fruits of your actions are not for your enjoyment. 3) Even while working, give up the pride of doer ship. 4) Do not be attached to inaction.

Do your duty, but do not concern yourself with the results. We have the right to do our duty, but the results are not dependent only upon our efforts. A few factors come into play in determining the results—our efforts, destiny (our past karmas), the will of God, the efforts of others, the cumulative karmas of the people involved, the place and situation (a matter of luck), etc. Now if we become anxious for results, we will experience anxiety whenever they are not according to our expectations. So, Krishna advises Arjun to give up concern for the results and instead focus solely on doing a good job. The fact is that when we are unconcerned about the results, we can focus entirely on our efforts, and the result is even better than before.

An interesting acronym for this is NATO or Not Attached to Outcome. Consider its application to a simple everyday activity such as playing golf. When people play golf, they are engrossed in the fruits—whether their shot has covered the right distance. Whether the score is under par, over par, etc.

Now if they could merely focus on playing the shots to the best of their ability, avoid the tendency to raise their head before completing the swing, they would find it as the most enjoyable game of golf they ever played. Additionally, with their complete focus on the shot being played, their game would be raised to a higher level.

The fruits of your actions are not for your enjoyment. To perform actions is an integral part of human nature. Having come into this world, we all have various duties determined by our family situation, social position, occupation, etc. While performing these actions, we must remember that we are not the enjoyers of the results—the results are meant for the pleasure of God. The individual soul is a tiny part of God (verse 15.7), and hence our inherent nature is to serve him through all our actions.

dāsa bhūtamidaṁ tasya jagatsthāvara jangamam
śhrīmannārāyaṇa swāmī jagatāṁprabhurīśhwaraḥ (Padma Puran) [v40]

"God is the Master of the entire creation; all moving and non-moving beings are his servants." Material consciousness is characterized by the following manner of thoughts, "I am the proprietor of all that I possess. It is all meant for my enjoyment. I have the right to enhance my possessions and maximize my enjoyment." The reverse of this is Spiritual consciousness, which is characterized by thoughts such as, "God is the owner and enjoyer of this entire world. I am merely his selfless servant. I must use all that I have in the service of God." Accordingly, Krishna instructs Arjun not to think of himself as the enjoyer of the fruits of his actions.

Ashtavakra Gita in chapter verse 6 makes the same statement.

dharmādharmau sukhaṃ duḥkhaṃ mānasāni na te bibho |
na kartā'si na bhoktā'si mukta evā'si sarvadā || 6 || CH 1

"Right or wrong, joy or sorrow
Do not affect you.
These are the attributes of the mind.
You are neither the doer, nor the enjoyer.
O the all-pervading one
You are ever free"

Even while working, give up the pride of doer ship. Krishna wants Arjun to give up *kartritwābhimān*, or the ego of being the doer. He instructs Arjun never to chase after preconceived motives attached to his actions nor consider himself as the cause of the results of his actions. However, we are often faced with this dilemma that when we perform actions, then why should we not consider ourselves as the doers of those actions? The reason is that our senses, mind, and intellect are inert; God energizes them with his power and puts them at our disposal. As a result, only with the help of the power we receive from him, are we able to work. For example, the tongs in the kitchen are inactive by themselves, but they get energized by someone's hand, and then they perform even difficult tasks, such as lifting burning coal, etc. Now if we think that the tongs are the doers of actions, it will be inaccurate. If the hand did not energize them, they will be unable to do anything. Similarly, if God does not supply our body-mind-soul mechanism with the power to perform actions, we would be incapable of doing anything. Thus, we must give up the ego of doing, remembering that God is the only source of the power by which we perform all our actions.

All the above thoughts are nicely summarized in the following popular Sanskrit verse:

yatkṛitaṁ yatkariṣhyāmi tatsarvaṁ na mayā kṛitam
tvayā kṛitaṁ tu phalabhuk tvameva madhusūdana [v41]

"Whatever I have achieved and whatever I wish to achieve, I am not the doer of these. O Madhusudan, you are the real doer, and you alone are the enjoyer of their results."

Do not be attached to inaction. Although the nature of the living being is to work, often situations arise where work seems burdensome and confusing. In such cases, instead of running away from it, we must understand and implement the proper science of work, as explained by Krishna to Arjun. However, it is highly inappropriate if we consider work as laborious and burdensome, and resort to inaction. Becoming attached to inaction is never the right solution.

Next two verses 48 and 49 of chapter 2 further reinforce the necessity of detachment to all actions and the results thereof. Maintaining perfect equanimity in all situations-regardless of fulfilment or non-fulfilment of goals is forcefully recommended. This is described as (समत्व भाव).

योगस्थ: कुरु कर्माणि सङ्गं त्यक्त्वा धनञ्जय |
सिद्ध्यसिद्ध्यो: समो भूत्वा समत्वं योग उच्यते || 48 || CH 2

yoga-sthaḥ kuru karmāṇi saṅgaṁ tyaktvā dhanañjaya
siddhy-asiddhyoḥ samo bhūtvā samatvaṁ yoga uchyate

yoga-sthaḥ—being steadfast in yog; kuru—perform; karmāṇi—duties; saṅgam—attachment; tyaktvā—having abandoned; dhanañjaya—Arjun; siddhi-asiddhyoḥ—in success and failure; samaḥ—equipoised; bhūtvā—becoming; samatvam—equanimity; yogaḥ—Yog; uchyate—is called

Translation

Be steadfast in the performance of your duty, O Arjun, abandoning attachment to success and failure. Such equanimity is called Yoga.

Commentary

The equanimity that enables us to accept all circumstances with serenity is so praiseworthy that Krishna calls it Yoga, or union with the Supreme. This equipoise comes from implementing the knowledge of the previous verse. When we understand that the effort is in our hands, not the results, we then concern ourselves only with doing our duty. The results are for the pleasure of God, and so we dedicate them to him. Now, if the results are not to our expectations, we calmly accept them as the will of God. In this way, we can accept fame and infamy, success and failure, pleasure and pain, as God's will, and when we learn to embrace both equally, we develop the equanimity that Krishna talks about.

The verse is a very practical solution to the vicissitudes of life. If we are sailing in the ocean in a boat, it is natural to expect the waves of the ocean to shake the boat. If we get disturbed each time a wave rocks the boat, our miseries would be endless. And if we do not expect the waves to arise, we would be expecting the ocean to become something other than its natural self. Waves are an inseparable phenomenon of the ocean. Similarly, as we wade through the ocean of life, it throws up all kinds of waves that are beyond our control. If we keep struggling to eliminate negative situations, we will be unable to avoid unhappiness. But if we can learn to accept everything that comes our way, without sacrificing our best efforts, we will have surrendered to the will of God, and that will be true Yoga.

दूरेण ह्यवरं कर्म बुद्धियोगाद्धनञ्जय |
बुद्धौ शरणमन्विच्छ कृपणा: फलहेतव: || 49 || CH 2

dūreṇa hy-avaraṁ karma buddhi-yogād dhanañjaya
buddhau śharaṇam anvichchha kṛipaṇāḥ phala-hetavaḥ

dūreṇa—(discrad) from far away; hi—certainly; avaram—inferior; karma—reward-seeking actions; buddhi-yogāt—with the intellect established in divine knowledge; dhanañjaya—Arjun; buddhau—divine knowledge and insight; śharaṇam—refuge; anvichchha—seek; kṛipaṇāḥ—miserly; phala-hetavaḥ—those seeking fruits of their work

Seek refuge in divine knowledge and insight, O Arjun, and discard reward-seeking actions that are certainly inferior to works performed with the intellect established in divine knowledge. Miserly are those who seek to enjoy the fruits of their works.

There are two aspects to work: 1) The external activity we do, 2) Our internal attitude toward it. For example, let us say that a temple is being built in the holy land of Vrindavan. The workers are engaged in a sacred activity, but their attitude is mundane. They are concerned with the salary they receive. If another contractor offers higher wages, they will not mind switching their job. There is also an ascetic living in Vrindavan, who, seeing the glorious temple being built, engages in *kār sevā* (voluntary work) as a service to God. The external work performed by the sadhu and the workers are the same, but the internal attitudes are poles apart.

Krishna advises Arjun to move higher in his internal motivation toward work. He declares that those who work with the motivation of self-enjoyment are miserly. Those who are detached from the fruits and dedicate their work to a higher cause are superior. And those who offer the fruits to God are truly in knowledge.

The word *kṛipaṇa* (miserly) has been used here. The Śhrīmad Bhāgavatam describes a *kṛipaṇa*:

na veda kṛipaṇaḥ śhreya ātmano guṇa-vastu-dṛik
tasya tān ichchhato yachchhed yadi so 'pi tathā-vidhaḥ (6.9.49) [v42]

"*Kṛipaṇa* are those who think that the ultimate reality consists only of sense objects produced from the material energy." Again, the Śhrīmad Bhāgavatam, states: *kṛipaṇo yo 'jitendriyaḥ* (11.19.44) [v43] "A *kṛipaṇa* is one who has no control over the senses."

As an individual evolves to higher levels of consciousness, one naturally sheds the desire for enjoying the fruits of work and moves in the direction of service. There are several examples of this nature in the historical and contemporary context.

Performance of all actions without any dependence on, or expectations of the reward is the most powerful message Krishna conveyed to the world at large. He advises complete absence of attachment to the action as well. Another message that is subsumed in these verses is perseverance in the performance of one's duties, regardless of the fact whether results are achieved or not, in line with one's expectations or otherwise. We often abandon work if results do not appear in accordance with our expectations. Sometimes we regard certain categories of work below our station and avoid doing them even if these are essential and are governed by our Dharma.

The emphasis is clearly on an uninterrupted performance of actions in accordance with one's Dharma without being judgemental about the quality or standard of work.

In our worldly existence, where material prosperity, power, wealth and recognition are regarded as the hallmark of success, following the philosophy and dictates of Karam Yoga pose a huge challenge. The usual refrain is that we work to earn name, fame, wealth and if there is no clarity with respect to reward, there is no motivation, and hence the quality of efforts required would be compromised. Reward and the quantum of reward operates as the biggest motivation and makes everyone put in that extra effort. This argument at the face of it may appear convincing, but a deeper analysis will make it clear that it is inherently flawed. Karam yoga never argues against accepting the reward of one's work, nor does it advocate renunciation or refusal of what is legitimately due. It only encourages everyone to focus on the work without being weighed down with the burden of rewards-how much, how soon. It is evident that, the rewards would be commensurate with the efforts and if our attention is on the reward, the quality of the efforts made would suffer. Adherence to the principles of Karam Yoga really improves the quality of our work and correspondingly, the quality and the quantum of rewards improves. Patience and perseverance in performance are the other attributes of Karam Yoga.

Everybody must keep working every moment of his existence and yet very often the desired rewards are not forthcoming. Sometimes, strong focus, intensive effort and hard work also do not yield the expected result. This can cause disillusionment and often leads people to abandon work or renounce the world. Here again to a question asked by Arjuna on the relative merits of renunciation and Karam yoga, Krishna categorically recommends Karam Yoga as a better option.

श्रीभगवानुवाच |
संन्यास: कर्मयोगश्च नि:श्रेयसकरावुभौ |
तयोस्तु कर्मसंन्यासात्कर्मयोगो विशिष्यते || 2 ||

śhrī bhagavān uvācha
sannyāsaḥ karma-yogaśh cha niḥśhreyasa-karāvubhau
tayos tu karma-sannyāsāt karma-yogo viśhiṣhyate

śhrī-bhagavān uvācha—the Supreme Lord said; sanyāsaḥ—renunciation; karma-yogaḥ—working in devotion; cha—and; niḥśhreyasa-karau—lead to the supreme goal; ubhau—both; tayoḥ—of the two; tu—but; karma-sanyāsāt—renunciation of actions; karma-yogaḥ—working in devotion; viśhiṣhyate—is superior

The Supreme Lord said: Both the path of *karma sanyās* (renunciation of actions) and *karma yoga* (working in devotion) lead to the supreme goal. But *karma yoga* is superior to *karma sanyās*.

Commentary

In this verse, Krishna compares *karma sanyās* and *karma-yoga*. It is a very deep verse; so, let's understand it one word at a time.

A *karm yogi* is one who does both, spiritual and social, duties. Social duties are done with the body while the mind is attached to God.

sochu mana yaha karm mama saba lakhata hari guru pyāre (Sādhan Bhakti Tattva)

"Dear one! Think always that all your actions are being observed by God and Guru." This is the *sādhanā* of *karm-yog*, by which we gradually elevate ourselves from bodily consciousness to spiritual consciousness.

Karm sanyās is for elevated souls, who have already risen beyond the bodily platform. A *karm sanyāsī* is one who discards social duties due to complete absorption in God and engages entirely in the performance of spiritual duties (devotional service to God). This sentiment of *karm sanyās* was nicely expressed by Lakshman, when Lord Ram asked him to fulfill his worldly duties:

more sabai eka tumha swāmī, dīnabandhu ura antarayāmī (Ramayan)

Lakshman said to Ram, "You are my Master, Father, Mother, Friend, and everything. I will only fulfil my duty toward You with all my might. So please do not tell me about any of my bodily duties."

Those who practice *karm sanyās* do not consider themselves to be the body, and as a result, they do not feel obligated to discharge their bodily duties. Such *karm sanyāsīs* dedicate their full time and energy to spirituality, while *karm yogis* must split their time between worldly and spiritual duties. The *karm sanyāsīs* can thus move much faster toward God, while the *karm yogis* are encumbered with social duties.

However, in this verse, Krishna extols *karm-yog* beyond *karm sanyās* and recommends it to Arjun as the preferred path. This is because *karm sanyāsīs* are exposed to a danger. If, having renounced their duties they cannot absorb their mind in God, they become miserable. In India, there are tens of thousands of such sadhus, who felt they were detached, and thus, renounced the world, but their mind was not yet attached to God. Consequently, they could not experience the divine bliss of the spiritual path. And so, although wearing the saffron clothes of mendicants, they indulge in grossly sinful activities and lose out all they may have achieved on their spiritual path. Only the ignorant mistake their sloth as detachment from the world.

On the other hand, *karm yogis* do both their worldly duties and spiritual practice. So, if their mind turns away from spirituality, at least they have their work to fall back upon. *Karm-yog* is thus the safer path for majority of the people, while *karm sanyās* is only to be pursued under the expert guidance of a Guru.

The tenets of Karam Yoga have strong relevance for people who profess to engage in public service. With the advent of democracy in a major part of the world, politics became an important area of doing service for the people. However, politicians elected by the people assumed positions of authority and instead of becoming servants of the society, they became masters wielding enormous powers. The age-old maxim-power corrupts, and absolute power corrupts absolutely-became a reality. The real power (de jure) lies with the people, but de facto, it was exercised by a chosen few. The servants have now become the rulers. The general perception about politicians, with a few exceptions have taken a nose-dive. Here was a great opportunity for a class of people to dedicate their lives to the cause of service to the electorate, in building the nations with ethical actions and practices. Alas, that really is not happening.

This is where the principles of Karam Yoga become relevant. In public domain there is an additional responsibility on the elected representatives to stay engaged in work, only for the service of people. Fruits of their actions do not belong to them. They are required to observe austerity, provide selfless service and become a role model for the community. Ironically, some of the richest in the world today are either politicians or those who have leveraged their political connections to amass huge fortunes, much of which is not by fair means.

The mandates of Karam Yoga are applicable to everyone, but it is imperative for people in the public service and indeed, to the entire political class the world over.

In the beginning of chapter 18 Krishna analyses the arguments by several wise people on the relative merits of Karam Yoga and abandoning all work. He makes a final pronouncement in favour of continuous performance of one's prescribed duties in all situations.

यज्ञदानतपःकर्म न त्याज्यं कार्यमेव तत् |
यज्ञो दानं तपश्चैव पावनानि मनीषिणाम् || 5 || CH 18

yajña-dāna-tapaḥ-karma na tyājyaṁ kāryam eva tat
yajño dānaṁ tapaśh chaiva pāvanāni manīṣhiṇām

yajña—sacrifice; dāna—charity; tapaḥ—penance; karma—actions; na—never; tyājyam—should be abandoned; kāryam eva—must certainly be performed; tat—that; yajñaḥ—sacrifice; dānam—charity; tapaḥ—penance; cha—and; eva—indeed; pāvanāni—purifying; manīṣhiṇām—for the wise

Translation

Actions based upon sacrifice, charity, and penance should never be abandoned; they must certainly be performed. Indeed, acts of sacrifice, charity, and penance are purifying even for those who are wise.

Commentary

Here, Krishna pronounces his verdict that we should never renounce actions which elevate us and are beneficial for humankind. Such actions, if performed in the state of complete awareness, do not bind us, instead they help us grow spiritually. Consider, for example, a caterpillar. To transform itself, it weaves a cocoon for its evolution and encages itself in it. Once it becomes a butterfly, it breaks open the cocoon and soars into the sky. Our position in the world is like this. Like the ugly caterpillar, we are presently attached to the world and bereft of noble qualities. As a part of our self-preparation and self-education, we need to perform actions that bring about the inner transformation we desire. *Yajña* (sacrifice), *dān* (charity), and *tapa* (penance) are acts that help in our spiritual evolution and growth. At times, it may seem that they are binding too, but they are like the caterpillar's cocoon. They melt our impurities, beautify us from within, and effectually help us break through the shackles of earthly life. Hence, Krishna instructs in this verse that such auspicious activities must never be abandoned. He now qualifies his statement by revealing the proper attitude with which they must be performed.

एतान्यपि तु कर्माणि सङ्गं त्यक्त्वा फलानि च |
कर्तव्यानीति मे पार्थ निश्चितं मतमुत्तमम् || 6 || CH 18

etāny api tu karmāṇi saṅgaṁ tyaktvā phalāni cha
kartavyānīti me pārtha niśhchitaṁ matam uttamam

etāni—these; api tu—must certainly be; karmāṇi—activities; saṅgam—attachment; tyaktvā—giving up; phalāni—rewards; cha—and; kartavyāni—should be done as duty; iti—such; me—my; pārtha—Arjun, the son of Pritha; niśhchitam—definite; matam—opinion; uttamam—supreme

Translation

These activities must be performed without attachment and expectation for rewards. This is My definite and supreme verdict, O Arjun.

Commentary

Acts of sacrifice, charity, and penance should be done in the state of devotion to the Supreme Lord. If that consciousness has not been attained, then they should verily be performed as a matter of duty, without desire for reward. A mother abandons her selfish joys to perform her duty to her offspring. She offers the milk in her breast to her baby and nourishes the baby. She does not lose by giving to the child, rather she fulfils her motherhood. Similarly, a cow grazes grass in the meadow all day long but yields the milk in her udder to her calf. The cow does not become any less by performing its duty; on the other hand, such people are held in greater respect. Because these activities are performed selflessly, they are viewed as sacred. Krishna states in this verse that the wise should perform auspicious and beneficial acts in the attitude of selflessness. He now explains the three kinds of renunciation in the following three verses.

नियतस्य तु सन्न्यासः कर्मणो नोपपद्यते |
मोहात्तस्य परित्यागस्तामसः परिकीर्तितः || 7 || CH 18

niyatasya tu sannyāsaḥ karmaṇo nopapadyate
mohāt tasya parityāgas tāmasaḥ parikīrtitaḥ

niyatasya—of prescribed duties; tu—but; sanyāsaḥ—renunciation; karmaṇaḥ—actions; na—never; upapadyate—to be performed; mohāt—deluded; tasya—of that; parityāgaḥ—renunciation; tāmasaḥ—in the mode of ignorance; parikīrtitaḥ—has been declared

Translation

Prescribed duties should never be renounced. Such deluded renunciation is said to be in the mode of ignorance.

Commentary

Renouncing prohibited actions and unrighteous actions is proper; renouncing desire for the rewards of actions is also proper; but renouncing prescribed duties is never proper. Prescribed duties help purify the mind and elevate it from *tamo guṇa* to *rajo guṇa* to *sattva guṇa*. Abandoning them is an erroneous display of foolishness. Krishna states that giving up prescribed duties in the name of renunciation is said to be in the mode of ignorance.

Having come in this world, we all have obligatory duties. Fulfilling them helps develop many qualities in an individual, such as responsibility, discipline of the mind and senses, tolerance of pain and hardships, etc. Abandoning them, out of ignorance, leads to the degradation of the soul. These obligatory duties vary according to one's level of consciousness. For an ordinary person, acts such as earning wealth with ethical means, taking care of the family, bathing, eating, etc. are prescribed duties. As one gets elevated, these obligatory duties change. For an elevated soul, sacrifice, charity, and penance are the duties.

दुःखमित्येव यत्कर्म कायक्लेशभयात्यजेत् ।
स कृत्वा राजसं त्यागं नैव त्यागफलं लभेत् || 8 || CH 18

duḥkham ity eva yat karma kāya-kleśha-bhayāt tyajet
sa kṛitvā rājasaṁ tyāgaṁ naiva tyāga-phalaṁ labhet

duḥkham—troublesome; iti—as; eva—indeed; yat—which; karma—duties; kāya—bodily; kleśha—discomfort; bhayāt—out of fear; tyajet—giving up; saḥ—they; kṛitvā—having done; rājasam—in the mode of passion; tyāgam—renunciation of desires for enjoying the fruits of actions; na—never; eva—certainly; tyāga—renunciation of desires for enjoying the fruits of actions; phalam—result; labhet—attain

Translation

To give up prescribed duties because they are troublesome or cause bodily discomfort is renunciation in the mode of passion. Such renunciation is never beneficial or elevating.

Commentary

To advance in life does not mean abandoning our responsibilities, instead it entails increasing them. Novice spiritualists often do not understand this truth. Wishing to avoid pain and taking an escapist attitude, they make spiritual aspiration a pretext for relinquishing their obligatory duties. However, life is never meant to be without burdens. Advanced *sādhaks* are not those who are undisturbed because they do nothing, on the contrary, they retain their peace despite upholding a huge burden placed upon their shoulders. Krishna declares in this verse that giving up duties because they are troublesome is renunciation in the mode of passion.

From the beginning, the *Bhagavad Gita* is a call for action. Arjun finds his duty unpleasant and bothersome and, as a result, wishes to run away. from the battlefield. Krishna calls this ignorance and weakness. He encourages Arjun to continue doing his duty, even though it may be unpleasant, while simultaneously bringing about an internal transformation within him. For this purpose, he enlightens Arjun with spiritual knowledge and helps him develop the eyes of wisdom. Having heard the Bhagavad-Gita, Arjun does not change his profession, but changes the consciousness he brings to bear upon his activities. Previously, the motive behind his work was to secure the kingdom of Hastinapur for his comfort and glory. Later, he continues to do his work, but as an act of devotion to God.

कार्यमित्येव यत्कर्म नियतं क्रियतेऽर्जुन ।
सङ्गं त्यक्त्वा फलं चैव स त्यागः सात्त्विको मतः || 9 || CH 18

kāryam ity eva yat karma niyataṁ kriyate 'rjuna
saṅgaṁ tyaktvā phalaṁ chaiva sa tyāgaḥ sāttviko mataḥ

kāryam—as a duty; iti—as; eva—indeed; yat—which; karma niyatam—obligatory actions; kriyate—are performed; arjuna—Arjun; saṅgam—attachment; tyaktvā—relinquishing; phalam—reward; cha—and; eva—certainly; saḥ—such; tyāgaḥ—renunciation of desires for enjoying the fruits of actions; sāttvikaḥ—in the mode of goodness; mataḥ—considered

Translation

When actions are undertaken in response to duty, and one relinquishes attachment to any reward, O Arjun, it is considered renunciation in goodness.

Commentary

Krishna now describes the superior kind of renunciation, where we continue to perform our obligatory duties, but give up attachment to the fruit of actions. He describes this as the highest kind of renunciation, which is situated in the mode of goodness (*sāttvic*).

Renunciation is necessary for spiritual attainment. But the problem is that people's understanding of renunciation is very shallow, and they consider it to be only the external abandonment of works. Such renunciation leads to hypocrisy in which, while externally donning the robes of a renunciant, one internally contemplates upon the objects of the senses. There are many sadhus in India who come in this category. They left the world with the noble intention of God-realization, but because the mind was not yet detached from the objects of their senses, their renunciation did not bestow the desired fruits. Consequently, they found their actions did not lead them to a higher spiritual life at all. The defect was in their sequence—they strove first for external renunciation and later for internal detachment. The instruction of this verse is to reverse the sequence—first develop internal detachment and then renounce externally.

that human body is structured in a manner that it must stay engaged in action all the time. Every action will inevitably lead to some result or reward. Real renunciate is the one who renounces the reward of the work and not the work.

न हि देहभृता शक्यं त्यक्तुं कर्माण्यशेषतः |
यस्तु कर्मफलत्यागी स त्यागीत्यभिधीयते || 11 || CH 18

na hi deha-bhṛitā śhakyaṁ tyaktuṁ karmāṇy aśheṣhataḥ
yas tu karma-phala-tyāgī sa tyāgīty abhidhīyate

Elaborating it further, Krishna says that one who does not renounce the reward of his work will be the recipient of the good, bad or the mixed effect of his karma, but the one who has renounced the reward does not get impacted by any of these factors. He is for ever free.

अनिष्टमिष्टं मिश्रं च त्रिविधं कर्मणः फलम् |
भवत्यत्यागिनां प्रेत्य न तु सन्न्यासिनां क्वचित् || 12 || CH 18

aniṣhṭam iṣhṭaṁ miśhraṁ cha tri-vidhaṁ karmaṇaḥ phalam
bhavaty atyāgināṁ pretya na tu sannyāsināṁ kvachit

While Karam Yoga should remain a preferred option, Gita throws light on the factors that are essential for a successful completion of any task. Verses 13, 14, 15 of chapter 18 are noteworthy. It is observed that there are five factors that are mandatory for any task to be completed in accordance with set goal. These are-an institution, a doer, several instruments of work, different sets of endeavours and finally providential support which also becomes favourable on account of the effects of Karma. Interestingly, all acts performed through thought, speech and action require the presence of these factors with respect to all kinds of Karma and their desired effect-good or bad. It is further clarified that in driving all these actions, soul or consciousness has no role to play.

पञ्चैतानि महाबाहो कारणानि निबोध मे |
साङ् ख्ये कृतान्ते प्रोक्तानि सिद्धये सर्वकर्मणाम् || 13 || CH 18

pañchaitāni mahā-bāho kāraṇāni nibodha me
sānkhye kṛitānte proktāni siddhaye sarva-karmaṇām

pañcha—five; etāni—these; mahā-bāho—mighty-armed one; kāraṇāni—causes; nibodha—listen; me—from me; sānkhye—of Sānkhya; kṛita-ante—stop reactions of karmas; proktāni—explains; siddhaye—for the accomplishment; sarva—all; karmaṇām—of karmas

Translation

O Arjun, now learn from Me about the five factors that have been mentioned for the accomplishment of all actions in the doctrine of *Sānkhya*, which explains how to stop the reactions of karmas.

Commentary

On knowing that work can be performed without attachment to the fruits, a natural question arises: "What constitutes action?" Krishna announces to Arjun that he is going to address this question now, as this knowledge will help develop detachment from the results of actions. Simultaneously, he clarifies that the description of the five limbs of action is not a new analysis, but what has previously been described in the *Sānkhya* philosophy as well. *Sānkhya* refers to the system of philosophy established by Maharishi Kapil, who was a descension of God and appeared on the earth as the child of Kardam Muni and Devahuti. The *Sānkhya* philosophy he propounded is based upon a system of analytical rationality. It develops knowledge of the self through an analysis of the elements within the body and in the world. It also ascertains the nature of cause and effect by an analysis of the elements of action. He is credited with establishing the laws of causality that govern all phenomena that take place in everyone's life.

अधिष्ठानं तथा कर्ता करणं च पृथग्विधम् |
विविधाश्च पृथक्चेष्टा दैवं चैवात्र पञ्चमम् || 14 || CH 18

adhiṣhṭhānaṁ tathā kartā karaṇaṁ cha pṛithag-vidham
vividhāśh cha pṛithak cheṣhṭā daivaṁ chaivātra pañchamam

adhiṣhṭhānam—the body; tathā—also; kartā—the doer (soul); karaṇam—senses; cha—and; pṛithak-vidham—various kinds; vividhāḥ—many; cha—and; pṛithak—distinct; cheṣhṭāḥ—efforts; daivam—Divine Providence; cha eva atra—these certainly are (causes); pañchamam—the fifth

Translation

The body, the doer (soul), the various senses, the many kinds of efforts, and Divine Providence—these are the five factors of action.

Commentary

In this verse, *adhiṣhṭhānam* means "place of residence," and refers to the body, since karmas can only be performed when the soul is situated in the body. *Kartā* means "the doer," and refers to the soul. Although the soul itself does not perform actions, it inspires the body-mind-intellect mechanism with the life force to act. Further, it identifies with their actions, due to the influence of the ego. Therefore, it is responsible for the actions performed by the body, and it is called both the knower and the doer.

The Praśhna Upaniṣhad states: *eṣha hi draṣhṭā spraṣhṭā śhrotā ghrātā rasayitā mantā boddhā kartā vijñānātmā puruṣhaḥ sa pare 'kṣhara ātmani saṁpratiṣhṭhate* (4.9) [v3]

"It is the soul that sees, touches, hears, feels, tastes, thinks, and comprehends. Thus, the soul is to be considered both—the knower and the doer of actions." The Brahma Sūtra also states: *jño 'ta eva* (2.3.18) [v4] "It is truly the soul that is the knower." Again, the Brahma Sūtra states: *kartā śhāstrārthavattvāt* (2.3.33) [v5] "The soul is the doer of actions, and this is confirmed by the scriptures." From the above quotations, the soul is also a factor in accomplishing actions.

The senses are instruments used for performing actions. Without the senses, the soul could not have experienced the sensations of taste, touch, sight, smell, or sound. There are also the five working senses—hands, legs, voice, genitals, and anus. It is with their help that the soul accomplishes various kinds of work. Thus, the senses are also listed as factors in accomplishing actions.

Despite all the instruments of action, if one does not put in effort, nothing is ever done. In fact, effort is so important that Chanakya Pandit states in his Neeti Sūtras: *utsāhavatāṁ śhatravopi vaśhībhavanti* [v6] "With sufficient effort, even poor destiny can be transformed into good fortune." *Nirutvāhād daivaṁ patita* [v7] "Without proper effort, even good destiny can be converted into misfortune." Therefore, *cheṣhṭhā* (effort) is another ingredient of action.

God is seated within the body of the living being as the witness. Based upon their past karmas, he also bestows different abilities to different people to perform actions. One may call this Divine Providence. For example, some people possess the acumen for earning huge amounts of wealth. Their acquaintances become astonished by their brilliant financial analysis of complex situations. They also seem to be lucky with the risks they take. This special intellect is granted to them by God. Similarly, others seem to have God-given talents in fields such as sports, music, art, literature, etc. It is God who bestows people these special abilities, in accordance with their past karmas. He also grants the results of the present karmas. Hence, he is listed as one of the factors responsible for action.

शरीरवाङ्मनोभिर्यत्कर्म प्रारभते नरः |
न्याय्यं वा विपरीतं वा पञ्चैते तस्य हेतवः || 15 || CH 18

तत्रैवं सति कर्तारमात्मानं केवलं तु यः |
पश्यत्यकृतबुद्धित्वान्न स पश्यति दुर्मतिः || 16 || CH 18

śharīra-vāṅ-manobhir yat karma prārabhate naraḥ
nyāyyaṁ vā viparītaṁ vā pañchaite tasya hetavaḥ
tatraivaṁ sati kartāram ātmānaṁ kevalaṁ tu yaḥ
paśhyaty akṛita-buddhitvān na sa paśhyati durmatiḥ

śharīra-vāk-manobhiḥ—with body, speech, or mind; yat—which; karma—action; prārabhate—performs; naraḥ—a person; nyāyyam—proper; vā—or; viparītam—improper; vā—or; pañcha—five; ete—these; tasya—their; hetavaḥ—factors; tatra—there; evam sati—in spite of this; kartāram—the doer; ātmānam—the soul; kevalam—only; tu—but; yaḥ—who; paśhyati—see; akṛita-buddhitvāt—with impure intellect; na—not; saḥ—they; paśhyati—see; durmatiḥ—foolish

Translation

These five are the contributory factors for whatever action is performed, whether proper or improper, with body, speech, or mind. Those who do not understand this regard the soul as the only doer. With their impure intellects they cannot see things as they are.

Commentary

The three kinds of actions are—*kāyik* (those performed with the body), *vāchik* (those performed by speech), and *mānasik* (those performed by the mind). In each of these categories, whether we do virtuous or sinful acts, the five causes mentioned in the previous verse are responsible. Due to the ego, we think of ourselves as the doers of our actions. "I achieved this." "I accomplished that." "I will do this." These are statements we make under the illusion of being the doer. Krishna's purpose in revealing this knowledge is to annihilate the soul's pride of doer ship. Thus, he states that those who see the soul only as the contributory factor for action do not see things as they truly are. If the soul were not granted a body by God, it could not have done anything at all. Further, if the body were not energized by God, it could have still done nothing. The Kenopaniṣhad states:

yadvāchānabhyuditaṁ yena vāgabhyudyate (1.4) [v8]

"*Brahman* cannot be described by the voice. By its inspiration, the voice gets the power to speak."

yanmanasā na manute yenāhurmano matam (1.5) [v9]

"*Brahman* cannot be understood by the mind and intellect. By its power, the mind and intellect work."

yachchakṣhuṣhā na paśhyati yena chakṣhūṁṣhi paśhyati (1.6) [v10]

"*Brahman* cannot be seen with the eyes. By its inspiration, the eyes see."

yachchhrotreṇa na śhṛiṇoti yena śhrotramidaṁ śhrutam (1.7) [v11]

"*Brahman* cannot be heard with the ears. By its power, the ears hear."

yat prāṇena na prāṇiti yena prāṇaḥ praṇīyate (1.8) [v12]

"*Brahman* cannot be energized by the life airs. By its inspiration, the life air's function."

This does not mean that the soul has no role in performing karmas. It is like the driver in the car, who controls the steering wheel of the car and decides where to turn it and at what speed to drive. Similarly, the soul too governs the actions of the body, mind, and intellect, but it should not claim credit for any action(s) for itself. If we see ourselves to be the sole cause of action, then we want to be the enjoyers of our actions as well. But when we free ourselves from the pride of doer ship and ascribe the credit of our efforts to the grace of God and the tools provided by him, then we realize that we are not the enjoyers of our actions, and all actions are an offering to Him. As explained in the next verse, this understanding helps us to dedicate to him every act of sacrifice, charity, and penance, and perform these with utmost dedication.

These three verses, 14,15 and 16 of chapter 18 make profound observations that has direct impact on successful achievements or non-completion of any task that we set for ourselves. In everything that we do, presence of all these five factors is essential. Absence of one factor alone can derail the entire process of pursuit of our goal. All of them, including Divine Providence become mandatory in achieving the desired results. Our endeavours, requisite instruments, expertise can all come to naught if the time is not favourable, or if the external environment is not conducive to completion of the task. The message is very clear and that emphasises the importance of perseverance and absolute commitment without worrying over when or how much reward would accrue out of our efforts in each task.

Decision to choose the quality and kind of karma to be performed must be taken judiciously and with well-considered thought. With minor cultural variations, everyone in the world everywhere, has a clear understanding of what is right or wrong, what is good or bad. There are some eternal truths that do not change with time or place. Speaking the truth, not hurting anybody wilfully, love for everybody, kindness, humility, gratitude, and shunning emotions like, hatred, jealousy, anger and greed are qualities and emotions that are universal in nature. All acts performed under such conditions are signs of a good human being and are respected everywhere.

It is extremely important to perform good deeds, because over a period these become an integral part of one's nature or character. Every act performed gives us an experience. And depending upon the quality of our experience either we repeat it or shun it. We develop related tendencies and over a time, these tendencies harden into our habits. Axiomatically, habits die hard, and these become an integral part of our nature. Verse 30 of chapter 13 is worth reading.

प्रकृत्यैव च कर्माणि क्रियमाणानि सर्वशः |
यः पश्यति तथात्मानमकर्तारं स पश्यति || 30 || CH 13

prakṛityaiva cha karmāṇi kriyamāṇāni sarvaśhaḥ
yaḥ paśhyati tathātmānam akartāraṁ sa paśhyati

prakṛityā—by material nature; eva—truly; cha—also; karmāṇi—actions; kriyamāṇāni—are performed; sarvaśhaḥ—all; yaḥ—who; paśhyati—see; tathā—also; ātmānam—(embodied) soul; akartāram—actionless; saḥ—they; paśhyati—see

Translation

They alone truly see who understand that all actions (of the body) are performed by material nature, while the embodied soul does nothing.

Commentary

The Tantra Bhāgavat states: *ahankārāt tu samsāro bhavet jīvasya na svataḥ* "The ego of being the body and the pride of being the doer trap the soul in the *samsara* of life and death." In material consciousness, the ego makes us identify with the body, and thus we attribute the actions of the body to the soul, and think, "I am doing this…I am doing that." But the enlightened soul perceives that while eating, drinking, talking, walking, etc. it is only the body that acts. Yet, it cannot shrug the responsibility of the actions performed by the body. Just as the President is responsible for the decision of the country to go to war, although he does not fight in it himself, similarly, the soul is responsible for the actions of a living entity, even though they are performed by the body, mind, and intellect. That is why a spiritual aspirant must keep both sides in mind. Maharishi Vasishth instructed Ram: *kartā bahirkartāntarloke vihara rāghava* (Yog Vāsiṣhṭh) "Ram, while working, externally exert Yourself as if the results depend upon You; but internally, realize Yourself to be the non-doer."

"Those who believe that it is one's material nature that drives all actions, and not the embodied soul, see the truth".

All our life we act strictly in accordance with our innate nature and our conduct largely becomes predictable. Most of our actions are performed in a state of unawareness and our sub-conscious becomes stronger than our conscious state.

Choose the right action and with due caution.
Weigh your words before delivering them.
Let our speech and action be preceded by thought and not the other way around.

Strict observance to the practice of Karam Yog is extremely difficult because of our inherent nature that wants to corner all the goods and glory for our benefit. We are essentially acquisitive and are driven not by need alone, but greed becomes the primary motive of our life. In contrast, animals lead a highly disciplined life, killing and eating only when, and what they need. The rich and powerful take a major share of the worlds' abundant resources and tend to store for many generations.

Our planet is amid an unprecedented crisis on account of massive ecological degradations, caused by reckless deforestation, pollution of the water bodies, exploitation of fossil resources for energy consumption and many other acts that have played havoc with environment. Carbon emissions, Ozone depletion is causing several health-related problems, leading to pandemics threatening lives of millions of people across all geographical regions. All this is symptomatic of the unbridled greed of a few nations and a few individuals, who have cornered massive spoils from the earth resources without allowing rejuvenation and restoration. Those who possess plenty are not satiated. They want more, even though they do not need it. Those who have little, or nothing are further deprived of the necessities. Data suggests that a quarter of century ago, the average disposable income of the richest 10% was around seven times higher than that of the poorest 10%. Now it is around 9.5 times higher. Evidently, this widening gap is hurting individuals, societies and even economies and is indeed unsustainable. Rather late in the day, United Nation after intensive deliberations involving several countries across the globe, adopted 17 goals to be achieved by 2030. These have been incorporated in a document titled "UN Sustainable development Goals". It sets a universal agenda for the entire world community with the following assertion.

"A path for the world in which prosperity is shared, societies are inclusive, and the environment is kept safe".

Vedanta through the instrumentality of several Upanishads has made very profound observations in this regard. Ishavasya Upanishad in second verse, makes the following statement.

ईशावास्यमिदं सर्वं यत्किञ्च जगत्यां जगत् ।
तेन त्यक्तेन भुञ्जीथा मा गृधः कस्यस्विद्धनम् ।।

Hindi meaning
जड़-चेतन प्राणियों वाली यह समस्त सृष्टि परमात्मा से व्याप्त है। मनुष्य इसके पदार्थों का आवश्यकतानुसार भोग करे, परंतु 'यह सब मेरा नहीं है के भाव के साथ' उनका संग्रह न करे।

English meaning
This universe, made of living and non-living things, is permeated by God. Humans may use the resources as needed but may not hoard as if 'this all belongs to me'.Message in this verse is clear and unambiguous. Everything that exists in the world-animate or inanimate, belongs to God. We may use it for our personal needs and not hoard it with any thought of personal ownership. In fact, spirituality promotes the concept of trusteeship. We are all trustees of material. Practice of Karam yoga alone can take you to a state of excellence.

Unencumbered by the expectation of reward, you can fully concentrate on you work and mission and give it your best. It promotes skills, develop expertise and deliver quality of work. Chapter 2 verse 50 makes a categorical statement in this regard.

बुद्धियुक्तो जहातीह उभे सुकृतदुष्कृते ।
तस्माद्योगाय युज्यस्व योगः कर्मसु कौशलम् || 50 || CH 2

buddhi-yukto jahātīha ubhe sukṛita-duṣhkṛite
tasmād yogāya yujyasva yogaḥ karmasu kauśhalam

buddhi-yuktah—endowed with wisdom; jahāti—get rid of; iha—in this life; ubhe—both; sukṛita-duṣhkṛite—good and bad deeds; tasmāt—therefore; yogāya—for Yog; yujyasva—strive for; yogaḥ—yog is; karmasu kauśhalam—the art of working skillfully

One who prudently practices the science of work without attachment can get rid of both good and bad reactions in this life itself. Therefore, strive for Yog, which is the art of working skilfully (in proper consciousness).

Observance of Karam Yoga has an equal validity in spiritual and temporal domains. It assures excellence in the material world and successfully takes you to your chosen goal. In the spiritual domain, if you work only for the sake of work and treat the reward as an offering to Him, you attain the goal of self-realisation. Krishna has raised the level of Karam Yoga well above knowledge and meditation. Chapter 12 verse 12

श्रेयो हि ज्ञानमभ्यासाज्ज्ञानाद्ध्यानं विशिष्यते ।
ध्यानात्कर्मफलत्यागस्त्यागाच्छान्तिरनन्तरम् || 12 || CH 12

śhreyo hi jñānam abhyāsāj jñānād dhyānaṁ viśhiṣhyate
dhyānāt karma-phala-tyāgas tyāgāch chhāntir anantaram

śhreyaḥ—better; hi—for; jñānam—knowledge; abhyāsāt—than (mechanical) practice; jñānāt—than knowledge; dhyānam—meditation; viśhiṣhyate—better; dhyānāt—than meditation; karma-phala-tyāgaḥ—renunciation of the fruits of actions; tyāgāt—renunciation; śhāntiḥ—peace; anantaram—immediately

Better than mechanical practice is knowledge; better than knowledge is meditation. Better than meditation is renunciation of the fruits of actions, for peace immediately follows such renunciation.

All great people in the world who have made seminal contribution to the upliftment of all and created sustainable benefits for society through their erudition, scientific breakthrough, medicine or in public or political domains (जन कल्याण), have been quintessentially Karma yogis. All acts performed by them are generally directed towards achieving public good which really amounts to an offering to God. They start with a mission, have clarity of goals, and pursue them with single minded devotion. Another interesting fact about such people is that, notwithstanding several impediments on their way, they never abandon the mission. Non-fulfilment of the task that they set for themselves, does not deter them from their chosen paths. There are moments of frustrations, failures, or slow progress in every mission, but a karma yogi would steadfastly persevere, and results usually are rewarding, sometime sooner than one expects.

Major scientific discoveries have been made by people across the world on the strength of Karma yoga. They spend a lifetime pursuing their goals, overcoming multiple challenges, moments of disappointment but never give up.

Practice of Karam yoga requires a sense of detachment verging on renunciation. Here renunciation does not signify giving up all material possessions or depriving oneself of necessities of life or head towards the forest or the hills. It simply means a sense of non-attachment, a kind of Vairagya towards worldly comforts and giving up on our inherently acquisitive nature.

Karam yoga is a kind of a mind-set and its practice supported by a firm belief leads us to a state of liberation. It sets us free. All of us must stay engaged in work all the time, and if we identify ourselves with the work and wait for the results that should follow, we get bound. Bondage of any kind is slavery and often is a cause of deep misery. Rewards of our work may sometime give us momentary happiness, but that is transient. Material possessions, success or fame are of a temporary nature. They come and go, and we alternate between moments of happiness and misery. Alternatively, a sense of detachment from the work and its rewards provides a sense of equanimity and in either situation, one remains unaffected.

Interestingly, a true karma yogi works with absolute commitment and dedication without being burdened with the thoughts of success or failure. He may appear to work with passion, but he is free, sanguine marked with dispassion. He has given up the notions of I, Me, Mine and Myself. These pronouns, either subjective or objective connote strong attachment to all actions and their results, and one starts identifying everything with the I as a subject. The following two verses help to disabuse any possibility of the soul acting as a doer.

प्रकृत्यैव च कर्माणि क्रियमाणानि सर्वशः |
यः पश्यति तथात्मानमकर्तारं स पश्यति || 29 || CH 13

prakṛityaiva cha karmāṇi kriyamāṇāni sarvaśhaḥ
yaḥ paśhyati tathātmānam akartāraṁ sa paśhyati

prakṛityā—by material nature; eva—truly; cha—also; karmāṇi—actions; kriyamāṇāni—are performed; sarvaśhaḥ—all; yaḥ—who; paśhyati—see; tathā—also; ātmānam—(embodied) soul; akartāram—actionless; saḥ—they; paśhyati—see

They alone truly see who understand that all actions (of the body) are performed by material nature, while the embodied soul does nothing.

प्रकृतेः क्रियमाणानि गुणैः कर्माणि सर्वशः |
अहङ्कारविमूढात्मा कर्ताहमिति मन्यते || 27 || CH 3

prakṛiteḥ kriyamāṇāni guṇaiḥ karmāṇi sarvaśhaḥ
ahankāra-vimūḍhātmā kartāham iti manyate

prakṛiteḥ—of material nature; kriyamāṇāni—carried out; guṇaiḥ—by the three modes; karmāṇi—activities; sarvaśhaḥ—all kinds of; ahankāra-vimūḍha-ātmā—those who are bewildered by the ego and misidentify themselves with the body; kartā—the doer; aham—I; iti—thus; manyate—thinks

All activities are carried out by the three modes of material nature. But in ignorance, the soul, deluded by false identification with the body, thinks of itself as the doer.

Practice of Karma yoga is antithetical to the concept of ownership of the material possessions including one's body-mind-intellect. Several philosophers and indeed, scientists, neuro-physicists the world over are engaged in a fierce debate over the issue of mind and matter. The classic quote doing the rounds is- 'Mind is no matter and matter, never mind'. Many thought leaders, especially in the west inspired by the Vedanta philosophy are attempting to create a synthesis between science and spirituality, and several impressions or myths associated with soul/consciousness are being revised. The difference between the two is getting blurred. This is leading to a better understanding of numerous phenomena hitherto unexplained in the field of science, especially Physics. One of the important branches of Yoga-Sankhya Yoga which takes a different view of the existence of Brahman as professed by the Advait Vedanta, mentions Prakriti and Purusha as two separate entities. Prakriti, another face of the cosmic nature has four distinct dimensions that impact the universe and all beings. These are-Time, Space, Matter and Energy. New research by the scientists is leading to certain propositions that will create a better understanding of the origin of universe and its evolutionary process.

Hans-Peter Duerr, Emeritus Professor of Max Planck Institute in Munich who succeeded Albert Einstein and Werner Heisenberg, mentions that Matter and energy are the two side of the same coin, they are not two distinct entities at the subtlest level. Trying to look at matter at its subtlest level for the past 55 years, Hans Peter realised that there is no matter distinct from energy at that level. That vast omnipotent energy is the universal consciousness (or God) and we humans are but a tiny bit of that consciousness, the individual consciousness.

He further adds rather cryptically, "Whenever I give a lecture on Quantum Physics, I feel I am talking on Vedanta. I studied matter for the last 35 years only to find out that it does not exist! I have been studying something that does not exist"-exactly what Adi Sankara said long back from the Upanishads.

Adi Shankaracharya does not dismiss the existence of matter per se. It is there for everyone to experience-the world with all in its material manifestations, but as a firm proponent of Advait Vedanta, he describes the world and the matter only as an appearance in our consciousness. According to him it is the consciousness or awareness alone that is real and illumines all that is seen or experienced by our body-mind-intellect. It is a witness unaffected by what is going on in the world.

ALL THAT YOU SEE DOES NOT EXIST

Ashtavakra Gita, the purest text on the ideology of Advaita Vedanta echoes similar view.

Verse 18 Chapter 1
aaakaaram anrutham viddhi niraakaaram thu nischalam ethath thathvopadeshen na punarbhava sambhava

Translation
Know that the form is unreal, but the formless is permanently stable. By the instruction of this fact, rebirth becomes impossible.

The foregoing statements, coupled with unambiguous observations by the leading scientists further underscore the relevance of Karam Yog. If matter does not exist and whatever is visible is unreal, then seeking it, possessing it with unbridled avarice is pointless. It is perishable, transient, and illusory. This is exactly Karam Yog is trying to emphasis upon-Why chase something that does not exist, or which is at best ephemeral. Work for the sake of work and not of the rewards thereof which in any case will not stay with you.

If the work is the only thing to focus on than it is important to analyse the kind of work that should be chosen.

श्रेयान्स्वधर्मो विगुण: परधर्मात्स्वनुष्ठितात् |
स्वधर्मे निधनं श्रेय: परधर्मो भयावह: || 35 || CH 3

śhreyān swa-dharmo viguṇaḥ para-dharmāt sv-anuṣhṭhitāt
swa-dharme nidhanaṁ śhreyaḥ para-dharmo bhayāvahaḥ

śhreyān—better; swa-dharmaḥ—personal duty; viguṇaḥ—tinged with faults; para-dharmāt—than another's prescribed duties; su-anuṣhṭhitāt—perfectly done; swa-dharme—in one's personal duties; nidhanam—death; śhreyaḥ—better; para-dharmaḥ—duties prescribed for others; bhaya-āvahaḥ—fraught with fear

It is far better to perform one's natural prescribed duty, though tinged with faults, than to perform another's prescribed duty, though perfectly. In fact, it is preferable to die in the discharge of one's duty, then to follow the path of another, which is fraught with danger.

In this verse, the word *dharma* has been used four times. *Dharma* is a word commonly used in Hinduism and Buddhism. But it is the most elusive word to translate into the English language. Terms like righteousness, good conduct, duty, noble quality, etc. only describe an aspect of its meaning. *Dharma* comes from the root word *dhṛi*, which means *ḍhāraṇ karane yogya*, or "responsibilities, duties, thoughts, and actions that are appropriate for us." For example, the dharma of the soul is to love God. It is like the central law of our being.

श्रेयान्स्वधर्मो विगुण: परधर्मात्स्वनुष्ठितात् ।
स्वभावनियतं कर्म कुर्वन्नाप्नोति किल्बिषम् ।। 47 ।। CH 18

śhreyān swa-dharmo viguṇaḥ para-dharmāt sv-anuṣhṭhitāt
svabhāva-niyataṁ karma kurvan nāpnoti kilbiṣham

śhreyān—better; swa-dharmaḥ—one's own prescribed occupational duty; viguṇaḥ—imperfectly done; para-dharmāt—than another's dharma; su-anuṣhṭhitāt—perfectly done; svabhāva-niyatam—according to one's innate nature; karma—duty; kurvan—by performing; na āpnoti—does not incur; kilbiṣham—sin

It is better to do one's own *dharma*, even though imperfectly, than to do another's *dharma*, even though perfectly. By doing one's innate duties, a person does not incur sin.

When we do our *swa-dharma* (prescribed occupational duties), there is a two-fold advantage. It is in tune with our disposition. Hence, it is as natural to our personality as flying is to a bird and swimming is to a fish. Secondly, since it is comfortable to the mind, it can almost be done involuntarily, and the consciousness becomes free to be engaged in devotion.

Instead, if we abandon our duties thinking them to be defective, and take up another's duties unsuitable for our nature, we struggle against the innate inclination of our personality. This was exactly Arjun's situation. His Kshatriya nature was inclined to military and administrative activities. Events drove him to a situation where it was necessary to participate in a war of righteousness. If he were to shirk from his duty and withdraw from the battlefield to practice austerities in the forest, it would not help him spiritually, for even in the forest, he would not be able to get away from his inherent nature. Likely, he would gather the tribal people in the jungle and become their king. Instead, it would be better for him to continue doing his duty born of his nature, and worship God by offering the fruits of his works to him.

When one becomes spiritually accomplished the *swa-dharma* changes. It no longer remains at the bodily platform; it becomes the *dharma* of the soul, which is devotion to God. At that stage, one is justified in giving up occupational duties and engaging wholeheartedly in devotion because that is now the *swa-dharma* of one's nature. For people with that eligibility, Krishna will give the conclusion in the end of the *Bhagavad Gita*: "Give up all varieties of *dharmas* and simply surrender unto me." (18.66) However, until that stage is reached, the instruction given in this verse applies.

Very often we are dissatisfied by the kind of work we do are assigned to do, in keeping with certain situations or our station in life. We must keep performing it with utmost commitment. No work is inferior, and our diligence can raise it to a level which can become an envy of others. Alternatively, perfection lies in the way we perform our assigned duties and there is nothing in this world that does not have some defects or imperfections. Krishna, on the quality of work that we all perform during different stages of our life says.

सहजं कर्म कौन्तेय सदोषमपि न त्यजेत् |
सर्वारम्भा हि दोषेण धूमेनाग्निरिवार्वता: || 48 || CH १८

सह-जम कर्म कौन्तेय स-दोषम अपि न त्यजेत
सर्वारम्भा हि दोषेण धूमनाग्निर इवावृता:

सह-जम् - स्वभाव से उत्पन्न ; कर्म - कर्तव्य ; कौन्तेय - कुंती के पुत्र अर्जुन ; स-दोषम् - दोषों के साथ ; –अपि भले ही ; –न त्यजेत् त्यागना नहीं चाहिए ; सर्व - आरम्भाः - सारे प्रयास ; – हिनिश्चय ही ; – दोषेणदुष्टता से ; – धूमेनधुएँ से ; अग्निः - अग्नि ; –इव के रूप में; आवृताः - ढका हुआ |

O son of Kunti (Arjuna), one should not abandon one's inborn duty, even though it has some imperfection, for all undertakings are marred by blemishes, as flame by smoke.

Several people develop a tendency to renounce the world and seek spiritual enlightenment. They move into places that assures them complete solitude by retiring to a secluded ashram, cave or head towards the mountains. However, they do not give up worldly desires or attachments. Taking to sannyasa without complete break from the material world and its offerings does not make them a yogi. In other words, you must practise karma yoga in all your dealings and thoughts to become eligible to be called a sanyasi. Physical distancing from home, family and material world is not enough to become a renunciate.

Observance of yoga in strict sense only entitles you to become a sanyasi. A mere abandonment of bodily activities without complete detachment from all worldly or material possessions-animate or inanimate does not make you either a yogi or a sanyasi. Krishna clarifies this position in the following two verses in chapter 6.

श्रीभगवानुवाच |
अनाश्रित: कर्मफलं कार्यं कर्म करोति य: |
स संन्यासी च योगी च न निरग्निर्न चाक्रिय: || 1 || CH 6

śhrī bhagavān uvācha
anāśhritaḥ karma-phalaṁ kāryaṁ karma karoti yaḥ
sa sannyāsī cha yogī cha na niragnir na chākriyaḥ

śhrī-bhagavān uvācha—the Supreme Lord said; anāśhritaḥ—not desiring; karma-phalam—results of actions; kāryam—obligatory; karma—work; karoti—perform; yaḥ—one who; saḥ—that person; sanyāsī—in the renounced order; cha—and; yogī—yogi; cha—and; na—not; niḥ—without; agniḥ—fire; na—not; cha—also; akriyaḥ—without activity

The Supreme Lord said: Those who perform prescribed duties without desiring the results of their actions are actual *sanyāsīs* (renunciates) and yogis, not those who have merely ceased performing sacrifices such as Agnihotra yajna or abandoned bodily activities.

The ritualistic activities described in the Vedas include fire sacrifices, such as Agnihotra yajna. The rules for those who enter the renounced order of *sanyās* state that they should not perform the ritualistic *karm kāṇḍ* activities; in fact, they should not touch fire at all, not even for the purpose of cooking. And they should subsist on alms instead. However, Krishna states in this verse that merely giving up the sacrificial fire does not make one a *sanyāsī* (renunciant).

Who are true yogis, and who are true *sanyāsīs*? There is much confusion in this regard. People say, "This swamiji is *phalāhārī* (one who eats only fruits and nothing else), and so he must be an elevated yogi." "This *bābājī* (renunciant) is *dūdhāhārī* (subsists on milk alone), and hence he must be an even higher yogi." "This guruji is *pavanāhārī* (does not eat, lives only on the breath), and so he must definitely be God-realized." "This sadhu is a *nāgā bābā* (ascetic who does not wear clothes), and thus he is perfectly renounced." However, Krishna dismisses all these concepts. He says that such external acts of asceticism do not make anyone either a *sanyāsī* or a yogi. Those who can renounce the fruits of their actions, by offering them to God, are the true renunciants and yogis.

Nowadays Yoga has become the buzz word in the western world. Numerous Yoga studios have sprung up in every town of every country of the world. Statistics reveal that one out of every ten persons in America is practicing Yoga. But this word "Yoga" does not exist in the Sanskrit scriptures. The actual word is "Yog," which means "union." It refers to the union of the individual consciousness with the divine consciousness. In other words, a yogi is one whose mind is fully absorbed in God. It also follows that such a yogi's mind is naturally detached from the world. Hence, the true yogi is also the true *sanyāsī*.

Persons who perform *Karm Yog* do all activities in the spirit of humble service to God without any desire whatsoever for rewards. Even though they may be *gṛihasthas* (living with a family), such persons are true yogis and the real renunciants.

कच्चिदेतच्छ्रुतं पार्थ त्वयैकाग्रेण चेतसा |
कच्चिदज्ञानसम्मोहः प्रनष्टस्ते धनञ्जय || 72 || CH 18

kachchid etach chhrutaṁ pārtha tvayaikāgreṇa chetasā
kachchid ajñāna-sammohaḥ pranaṣhṭas te dhanañjaya

kachchit—whether; etat—this; śhrutam—heard; pārtha—Arjun, the son of Pritha; tvayā—by you; eka-agreṇa chetasā—with a concentrated mind; kachchit—whether; ajñāna—ignorance; sammohaḥ—delusion; pranaṣhṭaḥ—destroyed; te—your; dhanañjaya—Arjun, conqueror of wealth

Translation

O Arjun, have you heard Me with a concentrated mind? Have your ignorance and delusion been destroyed?

Commentary

Krishna took the position of Arjun's teacher. It is natural for the teacher to inquire whether the student has grasped the subject or not. Krishna's intention of asking the question is that if Arjun has not understood, he is ready to re-explain or go into further details.

This is the last verse spoken by Krishna as it appears in Bhagavad-Gita.

In verse 63 of the same chapter, Krishna tells Arjuna that he has delivered on[e] of the most profound messages and indeed, knowledge to him. Now he mus[t] reflect on it and do what he thinks is right. Even at this stage, Krishna does n[ot] force him and gives him space and freedom to act the way Arjuna deems fit.

इति ते ज्ञानमाख्यातं गुह्याद्गुह्यतरं मया |
विमृश्यैतदशेषेण यथेच्छसि तथा कुरु || 63 || CH 18

iti te jñānam ākhyātaṁ guhyād guhyataraṁ mayā
vimṛiśhyaitad aśheṣheṇa yathechchhasi tathā kuru

iti—thus; te—to you; jñānam—knowledge; ākhyātam—explained; guhyāt—that secret knowledge; guhya-taram—still more secret knowledg[e]; mayā—by me; vimṛiśhya—pondering; etat—on this; aśheṣheṇa—completely; yathā—as; ichchhasi—you wish; tathā—so; kuru—do

Translation

Thus, I have explained to you this knowledge that is more secret than a[ll] secrets. Ponder over it deeply, and then do as you wish.

Commentary

A secret is that knowledge which is not accessible to majority of the peopl[e]. Most of the laws of Physics were a secret until a few centuries ago, and man[y] continue to remain so. Spiritual knowledge is profound and not realizabl[e] through direct perception. It needs to be learnt through the Guru and th[e] scriptures. Hence, it is described as secret. In the second chapter, Krishn[a] revealed knowledge of the soul, which is *guhya*, or secret knowledge. In th[e] seventh and eighth chapters, he explained knowledge of his powers, which i[s] *guhyatar*, or a bigger secret. In the ninth and subsequent chapters, he reveale[d] knowledge of his *bhakti*, which is *guhyatamam*, or the highest secret. In th[e] present chapter, verse 55, he revealed that he can be known in his persona[l] form only by *bhakti*. Krishna is now concluding the *Bhagavad Gita*. Havin[g] spoken the eighteen chapters, including most secret knowledge to Arjun, h[e] now leaves the choice in Arjun's hands. He says, "I have revealed to yo[u] profound and confidential knowledge. Now the choice is in your hands." Lor[d] Ram made a similar statement to the residents of Ayodhya.

He invited them all for his discourse:*eka bāra raghunātha bolāe, guru dwija purabāsī saba āe* (Ramayan) [v34]

"Once, Lord Ram called all the residents of Ayodhya. Everyone, including Guru Vasishth came to hear him." In the discourse, Lord Ram explained to them the purpose of human life and the way to accomplish it. In the end, he concluded:

nahiṅ anīti nahiṅ kachhu prabhutāī, sunahu karahu jo tumhahi sohāī
(Ramayan) [v35]

"The advice I have given to you is neither incorrect nor coercive. Listen to it carefully, contemplate over it, and then do what you wish."

This free will to choose between available alternatives has been given to the soul by God. The freedom of choice is not infinite. One cannot decide, "I choose to be the most intelligent person in the world." Our choices are limited by our past and present karmas. However, we do possess a certain amount of free will, for we are not machines in the hands of God. Sometimes people question that if God had not given us free will then we would not have done any evil. But then we would not have done anything good either. The opportunity to do good always comes with the danger of doing evil. More importantly, God wants us to love Him, and love is only possible when there is a choice. A machine cannot love for it does not have any freedom of choice. God created us with free will and provided us with choices so that we may choose him and thereby exercise our love for him. Even the all-powerful God cannot force an individual to love and surrender to Him; this decision must be made by the individual concerned. Here, Krishna is calling Arjun's attention to his free will and asking him to choose.

The paradigm of Sankhya Yoga points to the two parallel existence of Purusha and Prakriti. Prakriti is the tangible manifestation of God's creation and verily comprises four dimensions that impact the entire humanity, indeed the entire universe. These are-matter, time, space, and energy. The dimensions of matter and space are fixed and in a relative context remain immobile, Time and energy are ever flowing. The fifth dimension is **free will** which is available to everyone, and its usage governs our journey in this world, here, hereinafter, and beyond. This is closely intertwined with the law of karma. The exercise of free will, available to everyone is a unique proposition and determines our progress or regress in life. We are in this world surrounded by nature, environment, people, friends, power, and wealth, but when it comes to exercise them or relate to them, we are alone, and this is where free will becomes relevant.

In chapter 6, verse 5 and 6, Krishna makes an unambiguous statement in this regard.

उद्धरेदात्मनात्मानं नात्मानमवसादयेत् |
आत्मैव ह्यात्मनो बन्धुरात्मैव रिपुरात्मनः || 5 ||

uddhared ātmanātmānaṁ nātmānam avasādayet
ātmaiva hyātmano bandhur ātmaiva ripur ātmanaḥ

uddharet—elevate; ātmanā—through the mind; ātmānam—the self; na—not; ātmānam—the self; avasādayet—degrade; ātmā—the mind; eva—certainly; hi—indeed; ātmanaḥ—of the self; bandhuḥ—friend; ātmā—the mind; eva—certainly; ripuḥ—enemy; ātmanaḥ—of the self

Translation

Elevate yourself through the power of your mind, and not degrade yourself, for the mind can be the friend and the enemy of the self.

Commentary

We are responsible for our own elevation or debasement. Nobody can traverse the path of God-realization for us. Saints and Gurus show us the way, but we must travel it ourselves. There is a saying in Hindi: *ek peḍa do pakṣhī baiṭhe, ek guru ek chelā, apanī karanī guru utare, apanī karanī chelā*[v.01] "There are two birds sitting on a tree—one Guru and one disciple. The Guru will descend by his own works, and the disciple will also only be able to climb down by his own karmas."

We have had innumerable lifetimes before this one, and God-realized Saints were always present on Earth. At any period, if the world is devoid of such Saints, then the souls of that period cannot become God-realized. How then can they fulfil the purpose of human life, which is God-realization? Thus, God ensures that God-realized Saints are always present in every era, to guide the sincere seekers and inspire humanity. So, in infinite past lifetimes, many times we must have met God-realized Saints and yet we did not become God-realized. This means that the problem was not lack of proper guidance, but either our reticence in accepting it or working according to it. Thus, we must first accept responsibility for our present level of spirituality, or lack thereof. Only then will we gain the confidence that if we have brought ourselves to our present state, we can also elevate ourselves by our efforts.

When we suffer reversals on the path of spiritual growth, we tend to complain that others have caused havoc to us, and they are our enemies. However, our biggest enemy is our own mind. It is the saboteur that thwarts our aspirations for perfection. Shree Krishna states that, on the one hand, as the greatest benefactor of the soul the mind has the potential of giving us the most benefit; on the other hand, as our greatest adversary, it also has the potential for causing the maximum harm. A controlled mind can accomplish many beneficial endeavours, whereas an uncontrolled mind can degrade the consciousness with most ignoble thoughts.

To be able to use it as a friend, it is important to understand the mind's nature. Our mind operates at four levels:

Mind: When it creates thoughts, we call it *mana*, or the mind.

Intellect: When it analyses and decides, we call it *buddhi*, or intellect.

Chitta: When it gets attached to an object or person, we call it *chitta*.

Ego: When it identifies with the bodily identifications and becomes proud of things like wealth, status, beauty, and learning, we call it *ahankār*, or ego.

These are not four separate entities. They are simply four levels of functioning of the one mind. Hence, we may refer to them all together as the mind, or as the mind-intellect, or as the mind-intellect-ego, or as the mind-intellect-*chitta*-ego. They all refer to the same thing.

The use of the word ego here is different from its connotation in Freudian psychology. Sigmund Freud (1856 – 1939), an Austrian Psychologist/neurologist, proposed the first theory of psychology regarding how the mind works. According to him, the ego is the "real self" that bridges the gap between our untamed desires (Id) and the value system that is learnt during childhood (Superego).

Various scriptures describe the mind in one of these four ways for the purpose of explaining the concepts presented there. They are all referring to the same internal apparatus within us, which is together called *antaḥ karaṇ*, or the mind. For example:

The Pañchadaśhī refers to all four together as the mind, and states that it is the cause of material bondage.

In the *Bhagavad Gita*, Krishna repeatedly talks of the mind and the intellect as being two separate things and emphasizes the need to surrender both to God. The Yog Darśhan, while analyzing the different elements of nature, talks of three entities: mind, intellect, and ego.

Shankaracharya, while explaining the apparatus available to the soul, classifies the mind into four—mind, intellect, *chitta* and ego.

So, when Krishna says that we must use the mind to elevate the self, he means we must use the higher mind to elevate the lower mind. In other words, we must use the intellect to control the mind.

बन्धुरात्मात्मनस्तस्य येनात्मैवात्मना जितः |
अनात्मनस्तु शत्रुत्वे वर्तेतात्मैव शत्रुवत् || 6 ||

bandhur ātmātmanas tasya yenātmaivātmanā jitaḥ
anātmanas tu śhatrutve vartetātmaiva śhatru-vat

bandhuḥ—friend; ātmā—the mind; ātmanaḥ—for the person; tasya—of him; yena—by whom; ātmā—the mind; eva—certainly; ātmanā—for the person; jitaḥ—conquered; anātmanaḥ—of those with unconquered mind; tu—but; śhatrutve—for an enemy; varteta—remains; ātmā—the mind; eva—as; śhatru-vat—like an enemy

Translation

For those who have conquered the mind, it is their friend. For those who have failed to do so, the mind works like an enemy.

Commentary

We dissipate a large portion of our thought power and energy in combating people whom we perceive as enemies and potentially harmful to us. The Vedic scriptures say the biggest enemies—lust, anger, greed, envy, illusion, etc.—reside in our own mind. These internal enemies are even more pernicious than the outer ones. The external demons may injure us for some time, but the demons sitting within our own mind can make us live in constant wretchedness. We all know people who had everything favourable in the world, but lived miserable lives because their own mind tormented them incessantly through depression, hatred, tension, anxiety, and stress.

The Vedic philosophy lays great emphasis on the ramification of thoughts. Illness is not only caused by viruses and bacteria, but also by the negativities we harbour in the mind. If someone accidentally throws a stone at you, it may hurt for a few minutes, but by the next day, you will probably have forgotten about it. However, if someone says something unpleasant, it may continue to agitate your mind for years. This is the immense power of the thoughts. In the Buddhist scripture, the Dhammapada (1.3), the Buddha also expresses this truth vividly:

"I have been insulted! I have been hurt! I have been beaten! I have been robbed! Misery does not cease in those who harbour such thoughts.

When we nourish hatred in our mind, our negative thoughts do more damage to us than the object of our hatred. It has been very sagaciously stated: "Resentment is like drinking poison and hoping that the other person dies." The problem is that most people do not even realize that their own uncontrolled mind is causing them so much harm. Hence, the advice:

mana ko mano shatru usaki sunahu jani kachhu pyare (Sadhan Bhakti Tattva)[v1]

"Dear spiritual aspirant, look on your uncontrolled mind as your enemy. Do not come under its sway."

However, the same mind has the potential of becoming our best friend, if we bring it under control of the intellect, through spiritual practice. The more powerful an entity is, the greater is the danger of its misuse, and the greater is the scope for its utilization. Since the mind is such a powerful machine fitted into our bodies, it can work as a two-edged sword. Thus, those who slide to demoniac levels do so because of their own mind while those who attain sublime heights also do so because of their purified minds. Accordingly, Franklin D. Roosevelt, former President of America, expressed this very nicely: "Men are not prisoners of fate, but only prisoners of their own minds." In this verse, Krishna enlightens Arjun about the potential harm and benefits our mind can bestow upon us.

This is a great lesson in developing a strong leadership style. The leader must guide his followers, explain the pros and cons of a situation, empower them, and desist from forcing them. When you are empowered, you own that decision and put all your own efforts in achieving the task that has been set for you.

Karam yoga helps to create equilibrium and equanimity. You can se everything with a sense of detachment. You perform all duties with utmos dedication, indeed passion but do not get overwhelmed because rewards don bother you. You stay afloat and do not get drowned in the sea of materiality.

ब्रह्मण्याधाय कर्माणि सङ्गं त्यक्त्वा करोति यः |
लिप्यते न स पापेन पद्मपत्रमिवाम्भसा || 10 || CH 5

ब्राह्मणी - भगवान को ; आधाय– समर्पित करते हुए ; कर्माणि– समस्त कर्म ; संगम आसक्ति ; _ त्यक्त्वा– त्याग कर ; करोति– करता है ; यः– कौन ; _ लिप्यते - प्रभावि होता है ; न– कभी नहीं ; सः - वह व्यक्ति ; पापेन– पाप से ; पद्म-पत्रम् - कमल का पत्ता इवा- जैसे ; अम्बासा– जल से |

जो लोग अपने कार्यों को भगवान को समर्पित करते हैं, सभी आसक्ति को त्याग कर पाप से अछूते रहते हैं, जैसे कमल का पत्ता पानी से अछूता रहता है।

Citing the example of Lotus, Krishna says lead your life like a lotus flower tha grows and blossoms in a pond full of impurities that do not even touch it. I looks beautiful, emits fragrance and its stem provides sustenance to many.

Religion and spirituality have influenced the humanity and has been a integral part of mankind since inception. All societies, regardless of th geography, colour, creed, gender, or race have been subjected to the all pervading presence of religion. It has produced, atheists, agnostics and theist and have also given rise to syncretism. Religious organizations have als wielded immense powers on the subject and have used the instrument of fea to tame its followers. Christianity, for example dubbed the atheists as heretic and put many including great thought leaders and scientists to death in th name of religion. Islam also treats the non-believers as Kafir and recommend death as an essential part of the edicts of Koran. Fortunately, some religiou traditions of the East, such as Hinduism, Buddhism, Jainism have been mor tolerant of those who disagreed with it or refused to follow the dictates of th organized institutions.

Modern societies, however, have been more progressive in allowing greate freedom to people in following their chosen faith, largely because of th process of democratic evolution and secular thoughts taking centre-stage Inter-religious conversions frowned upon earlier are also quite common. B that as it may, every religious group likes to maintain its influence and indeed makes effort to expand and keep their flock together. Many methods are used including violence to achieve this. It is in number that they draw their power and wealth from and would loathe to loosen their grip.

While religious groups and many sects have mushroomed over the years giving them power and authority over their subjects, several malpractices have also inevitably crept in, causing irreparable damage to the cause of faith which is an essential attribute of a civilized society. Religions, the world over historically, have played a divisive role and have only jeopardised the mandates of establishing harmony in the world. Religions do not propagate the message of वसुधैव कुटुम्बकम. ((The entire world is one family). Religions create their own families and constantly work towards increasing the numbers. Inter religious conversions have been very common and have also been a cause of avoidable strife. The strategy of the religious groups has been to target societies where pernicious caste system has been creating unequal social strata. The members of the lower caste are evidently more vulnerable and if they are promised equality and other benefits, they are quick to convert. Religions prefer to keep their flock together, however small, tend to increase their numbers and draw their validity and sustenance on keeping them on the margin of real spirituality.

While a large majority of people inhabiting this planet owe allegiance to one religious faith or another, very few evolve to the higher level of spiritual achievements.

**मनुष्याणां सहस्रेषु कश्चिद्यतति सिद्धये |
यततामपि सिद्धानां कश्चिन्मां वेत्ति तत्त्वतः || 3 || CH 7**

*manuṣhyāṇāṁ sahasreṣhu kaśhchid yatati siddhaye
yatatām api siddhānāṁ kaśhchin māṁ vetti tattvataḥ*

manuṣhyāṇām—of men; sahasreṣhu—out of many thousands; kaśhchit—someone; yatati—strives; siddhaye—for perfection; yatatām—of those who strive; api—even; siddhānām—of those who have achieved perfection; kaśhchit—someone; mām—me; vetti—knows; tattvataḥ—in truth

Amongst thousands of persons, hardly one strives for perfection; and amongst those who have achieved perfection, hardly one knows Me in truth.

The word *siddhi* has numerous connotations and meanings. As per the Sanskrit dictionary, a few of them are attainment of supernatural power, accomplishment, success, performance, fulfilment, solution of a problem, completion of cooking or a task, healing, hitting the mark, maturing, supreme felicity, beatitude, an unusual skill or faculty, perfection.

In this verse, Krishna has used *siddhi* for perfection in the spiritual path. He says, "Only a tiny portion of the innumerable souls are fortunate to get a human birth. Amongst them, only a minuscule strive for spiritual perfection. And even among those perfected souls, ones who are aware of My divine glories and paramount position are very rare."

How is it that even perfected souls are unable to know God? The reason is without bhakti or loving devotion, it is not possible to realize the Supreme. Spiritual aspirants of *karm, jñāna, haṭha yog,* etc., cannot know God unless they include devotion in their practice. Shree Krishna has stated this fact several times in the Bhagavad Gita:

"The Supreme Divine Personality is greater than all that exists. Although He is all-pervading and all living beings are situated in Him, yet He can be known only through devotion." BG 8.22.

"O Arjun, by unalloyed devotion alone can I be known as I am, standing before you. Thereby, on receiving my divine vision, O scorcher of foes, one can enter union with me." BG 11.54
"Only by loving devotion to me does one come to know who I am in truth. Then, having come to know me, my devotee enters full consciousness of me." BG 18.55

Therefore, such spiritual aspirants who do not include devotion in their sadhana attain only limited theoretical knowledge or *jñāna*. And devoid of *vijñāna* the experiential knowledge, they are unable to know God or the Absolute Truth.

It would be worthwhile to examine why a large multitude of humanity is not able to raise their spiritual quotient and continue to operate at the fringes of spirituality. Let us test this phenomenon in the context of the tenets of Karam yoga. The principal characteristics of Karam yoga is selflessness, in worldly acquisitions, in service and in receipt of rewards of one's work. Indeed, a Karam yogi is completely detached to materiality of every kind. He may possess huge wealth and power but is not attached to them. Whether it stays or goes away, is of no concern to him. A Karam yogi is a renunciate at heart. This really is the main challenge for a spiritual seeker. Majority of mankind is extremely keen to move to higher levels of religious or spiritual space but finds it extremely difficult to let go the worldly possessions, earned, and acquired with enormous hard work overtime. Sense of fear, deep insecurity and continuous dependence on the worldly support makes him weak. There is also confusion about one's goal in life. If you limit yourself to the achievements of success in the world, in acquiring money, power and recognition, it becomes difficult, indeed impossible to follow the path of Karam yoga.

Path of spirituality conjures up a vision of a path of inherent goodness, values, ethics, and eventual journey that must lead to God realization. Interestingly, all of us wish to tread this path, but are afraid of doing so. All of us without a single exception, want to be good, perform good deeds and wish to be recognized as one. No one wants to become a bad person. No one wants to be called a bad person, but some knowingly or unknowingly perform certain acts that are universally placed in the category of bad acts. There is an example of Durodhyana in Mahabharata whose acts of omission and commission led to the greatest war in the mythological history of India.

Both sides, Kauravas and Pandavas had reconciled to the inevitability of war. Krishna, as a last-ditch effort to avert the war, approached Durodhyana to give away a small part of the kingdom that rightly fell towards the share of Pandavas. The story goes that Krishna mentioned to Durodhyana that by refusing to part with the legitimate share of Pandavas, he was not doing the right thing. Duryodhyana replied saying that please don't tell me what is right or what is wrong. I know it and I also know that what I am doing is not right. He outrightly refused, saying that he knew what he was doing was wrong, but he did not feel like doing the right things.

It may be an extreme example of wilful cussedness, but in normal times most of us lesser mortals are prone to follow this path at some point in life. Everyone agrees that Spirituality is a desirable path and is designed to create a society where everyone lives in perfect harmony with each other and indeed, with all living beings and the universe. It creates complete equilibrium and ensures that everyone is treated at par with equal rights to live a happy life.

A person who becomes spiritual is expected to be good, speak the truth always, not hurt any living being, not lose anger, is not given to avarice, nurtures limited desires. On the positive side, he must live a life of austerity, engage in selfless service, consistently perform acts of philanthropy and work for the general welfare of society, without any expectations of rewards for himself.

Let us pause here for a while and reflect on the probability of numbers who would willingly follow this path. A large multitude of people will agree with the desirability of such acts, perhaps happily perform them on a one-off basis, but doing them all the time with complete sense of commitment and sustainability poses a formidable challenge. A common refrain is about us being human, with responsibilities to our family and numerous desires that never seem fully fulfilled. Spirituality to them seems to involve giving up on several material possessions earned with a lot of hard work. Also, it may close doors to amassing wealth in future and being deprived of a life of comfort they are accustomed to. It is the fear of losing out that creates this psychosis.

This fear is essentially unfounded. Fundamentally, our personal needs are not very large. How much does a human being need to keep the body and soul together. More than the need, it is greed that drives are actions, coupled with a deep sense of insecurity for self and the family. Desire for acquisition of power and recognition does not let us rest and we keep wandering aimlessly, chasing a mirage that is non-existent or is elusive. All that is ephemeral and is antithetical to our existence that is eternal.

The path of spirituality insulates us from suffering that will inevitably happen in our life's journey, brings in immersive positivity in our behaviour and ensures sustainable happiness. We are not dependent on the material world for achieving them.

The path of religiosity in contrast to spirituality, seems more doable and easier. Spirituality is a tough call and as we move up the ladder, it becomes more demanding, more stringent. It requires control, discipline, abstinence, and a bit of renunciation. Renunciation not in the form of giving up the world or becoming a monk, but in minimizing one's needs and desires to a bare minimum. It also insists on a deep and a growing sense of detachment to the material comforts and other forms of gratification. Beyond a point, a spiritual person seeks enlightenment by transcending his ego and realizing the “Self”.

It would be interesting to pick up a quote from a famous French philosopher Teilhard de Chardin, who was also a palaeontologist and Jesuit priest.
“We are not human beings having a spiritual experience; we are spiritual beings having a human experience.”

The entire spiritual psychology is founded on this principle. We are not human beings striving to be spiritual; we are already spiritual.

However, our physical experience is so overwhelming that we forget our identity. But the substratum of our spiritual quotient survives, and we chose to become religious, a definite dilution of our core. Religion is less rigorous, less demanding and helps to create a quasi but a false sense of spirituality. We then draw solace from the fact that we have not abandoned the path of God or universal consciousness altogether. We perform worship on a routine and ritualistic basis, visit places of pilgrimage, and do some charity on special occasions. In brief, we become good albeit for a short interregnum. We are now ready to plunge into the daily humdrum doing all that we are accustomed to. Paradoxically, we become more tolerant of our imperfections and less of the those belonging to other religions. This creates conflicts that inevitably arise out of "I" and "You", "Us" and "Them" syndrome.

As swami Vivekananda mentioned- "All human beings are potentially divine". It is essential to convert this divinity into a kinetic mode and manifest it in our daily life.

We must humanize our relationship with divinity and indeed, divinize our relationship with humanity. That is the true test of abiding spirituality.

This is possible if we are spiritually grounded. And paradigm of Karam Yog is the most powerful means for most of us, who lead an active life with challenges that are inevitably thrown at us.

Renunciation of worldly desires in totality, not merely in words but in conduct and conviction alone makes you eligible to become a Karam yogi and raise your spiritual connect.

Benefits of Karam yoga

The most celebrated message of Bhagwadgita, Karam yoga takes you to the highest levels of temporal and spiritual achievements. Absolute focus and commitment to one's duty and work, unencumbered by any expectations of reward ensures excellence.

Loss or gain, victory or defeat do not matter. You remain sanguine and unruffled in all conditions.

You remain perpetually in a state of peace, happiness, and bliss. This indeed is our identity.

You become an asset to the society and can contribute to the overall growth and development in a selfless manner.

A deep sense of detachment keeps you insulated from any worldly grief or misery.

You have no fear of losing anything and can perform all your work fearlessly act fearlessly.

A Karam yogi commands respect in all domains.

Selflessness and unselfish behaviour are the hallmark of a Karma Yogi.

One of the greatest advantages of following the path of Karam Yoga is the removal of impurities of our heart and mind. These impurities are caused primarily by several worldly desires that we accumulate over lifetime. Each one of us represents a bundle of desires that never seem to end. This becomes the biggest hindrance to acquisition of true knowledge. Karam Yoga is a great purifier.

If at any stage of one's life, driven by a phenomenon of anagnorisis, one realises that one has been living only for oneself, has not done anything for others, society, or the universe, take to Karma Yoga.

All great personalities in all domains, who have achieved something of value for the society, and are remembered for generations have been Karma Yogis.

CHAPTER FOUR

RAJA YOGA DHYAN YOGA

Yoga in everyone's life.

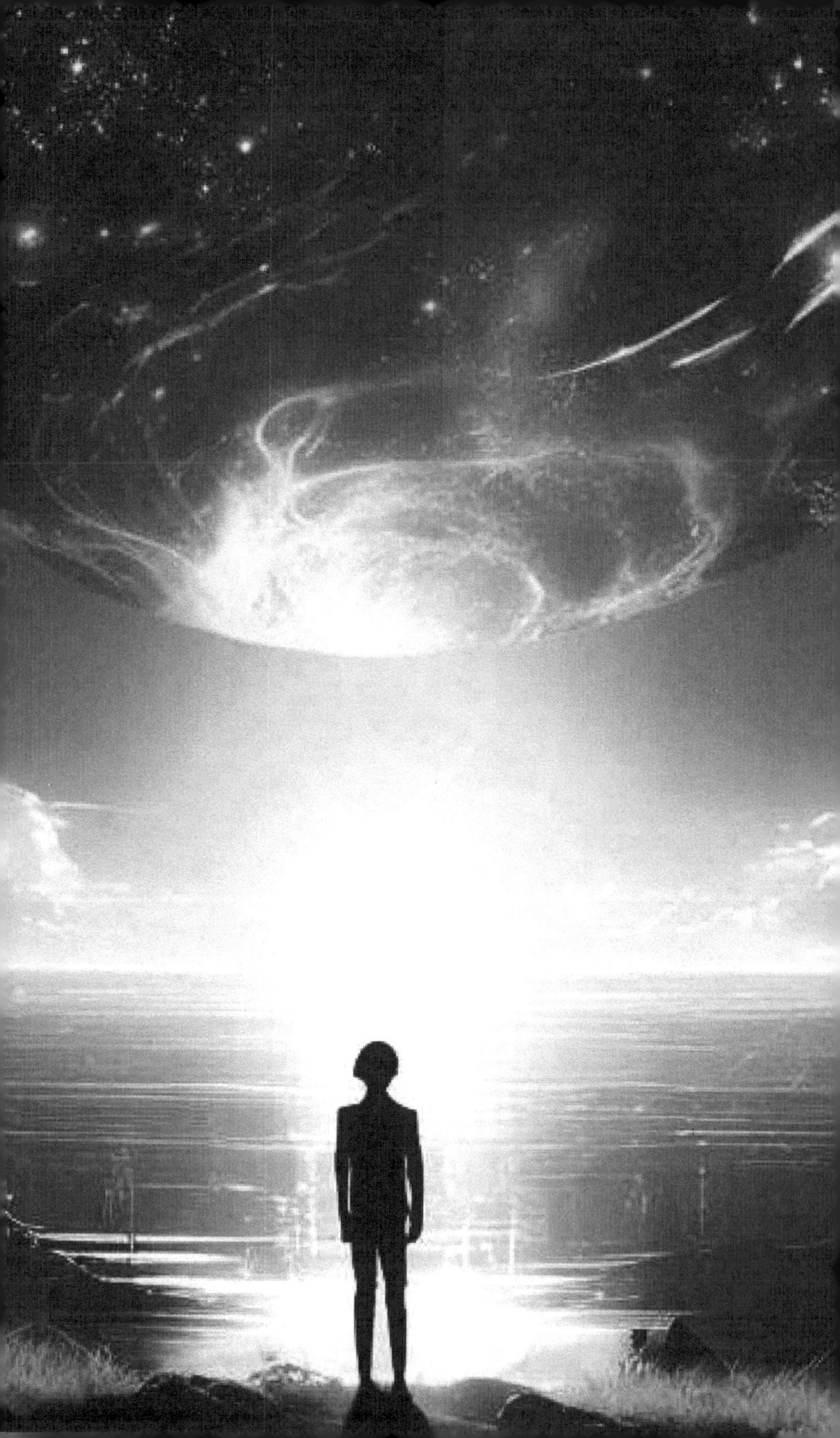

RAJA YOGA
DHYAN YOGA

There are several paradigms of Yoga being practised by its followers and each one of them creates benefits consistent with our state of mind and movement in our spiritual journey. Those in love with their God follow the path of Bhakti yoga and problems arising of lack of faith are addressed. Those who are inspired by a spirit of selflessness and detachment to the worldly issues, take to Karma yoga. There is a large section of humanity whose mind is restless, cannot focus and suffer from uncertainties of life-the remedy is Raja yoga or Dhyana Yoga. The methods in this form of yoga look like the current practice of mindfulness, but also create benefits for both mind and body. Majority of mankind has a limited perspective of their existence-limited to mind and body. This perhaps is the reason why Raja yoga has caught the imagination of people worldwide and is hence, the most prevalent form amongst several other forms that are designed to provide comprehensive advantages to mind-body-soul.

Our mind and intellect are at the core of our existence and drive all our actions. It is here that our thoughts and desire emerge. All our life's experiences and subsequent behaviour find their momentum from here.

Maitri Upanishad makes the following observation:

"One's own thought is one's world. What a person thinks is what he becomes".

A look at any being human, including self, combined by our own experience will reveal our gross/subtle possessions functioning in a hierarchical structure.

इन्द्रियाणि पराण्याहुरिन्द्रियेभ्य: परं मन: |
मनसस्तु परा बुद्धिर्यो बुद्धे: परतस्तु स: || 42||CH 3

indriyāṇi parāṇyāhur indriyebhyaḥ paraṁ manaḥ
manasas tu parā buddhir yo buddheḥ paratas tu saḥ

indriyāṇi—senses; parāṇi—superior; āhuḥ—are said; indriyebhyaḥ—than the senses; param—superior; manaḥ—the mind; manasaḥ—than the mind; tu—but; parā—superior; buddhiḥ—intellect; yaḥ—who; buddheḥ—than the intellect; parataḥ—more superior; tu—but; saḥ—that (soul)

The senses are superior to the gross body, and superior to the senses is the mind. Beyond the mind is the intellect, and even beyond the intellect is the soul.

An inferior entity can be controlled by its superior entity. Krishna explains the gradation of superiority amongst the instruments God has provided to us. He describes that the body is made of gross matter; superior to it are the five knowledge-bearing senses (which grasp the perceptions of taste, touch, sight, smell, and sound); beyond the senses is the mind; superior to the mind is the intellect, with its ability to discriminate; but even beyond the intellect is the divine soul.

This knowledge of the sequence of superiority amongst the senses, mind, intellect, and soul, can give us a clear understanding of our identity. However, it must be observed that amongst all instruments available to us only the body is gross. All other instruments are subtle in nature. Sense organs have a symbolic presence, but their experiences are subtle and hence vary from one individual to another. These experiences cannot be standardised. Similarly, all of us are aware of the existence of mind and intellect which are only perceptive. We do not need to mix them up with brain and heart that are goss manifestation of their subtle and personalized functionality.

The current practice of Raja yoga draws its origin from one of the very ancient scriptures known as **Yoga Sutra,** written by Maharishi Patanjali. It is also known as **Ashtanga Yoga** because of eight independent components, and each one of them must be mastered/practised to achieve an ultimate state of Samadhi which marks the culmination of this paradigm. Yoga Sutra is divided in four chapters and contains 195 aphorisms-51, 55, 56 and 33 respectively. First chapter shows the way to Concentration and its spiritual usage, the second one talks about Concentration and its practice. Third chapter comprehensively delineates the Yoga powers and fourth the last one, creates freedom and absorption.

The primary focus of Raja Yoga is on the study of human mind and seeks to create a state of thoughtless consciousness by observing its general tendencies and modifications. Transcending identification with mind-body-intellect and making pure consciousness as the core of human existence, it helps to calm and stabilize the mind. Methodology recommended to achieve this is-Meditation or in Sanskrit, Dhyana. Raja Yoga is essentially a Psycho-physical paradigm with a prevalence on the psychological structure of our being.

Raja yoga has extensively derived from Samkhya yoga, which is essentially dualistic in nature, in contrast to the Advaita philosophy propounded by Adi Shankaracharya, that recognises Brahman as the only entity and everything though its manifestation, is illusory.

ब्रह्म सत्यम जगत मिथ्या जीवो ब्रह्मैव ना अपरहा

Literally translated it means that Brahman alone is real, and Jagat is false, and the Jiva is non-different from Brahman.

For better appreciation of the science of Raja Yoga we will have to look at the tenets of Samkhya Yoga which recognises two entities-**Purusha and Prakriti**. The entire universe operates, based on a constant interplay of these two entities. It is believed that sage Kapila, who lived about 5000 years ago was the father of Samkhya philosophy. He is also hailed as the first philosopher of human race. Kapila is also credited with introducing the laws of causality which provide the scientific basis for Karmic philosophy. All experiences gained by Purusha which is gender-agnostic are possible with the presence and help of Prakriti, which really means the entire nature, the material world and everything that stays in the bosom of nature-gross or subtle. Independent of Prakriti, Purusha which is recognized as pure consciousness in both Advaita and Samkhya, cannot have any experience. Every experience comprises purusha and prakriti; subject and the object; consciousness and nature. Advaita Vedanta propagates the concept of only one Brahman and everything else including Prakriti as Maya, an illusion which does not exist or at best has an existence which is ephemeral. It appears to exist but is non-eternal and transient. It is like an appearance that human beings experience in dream state. As soon as we regain our awakened state, it disappears and only Purusha-the pure consciousness remains. While the approach in two paradigms is slightly different, the difference from the perspectives of the practice of Raja Yoga is only one of semantics.

As mentioned earlier, Patañjali divided his *Yoga Sutras* into four chapters or books (Sanskrit *Pada*), containing in all 195 aphorisms, divided as follows:

The first sutra is a formal announcement of the beginning of the formal text and reads.

Ath Yoga anushasanam

Now Yoga Discipline is explained.

Samadhi Pada

Samadhi Pada (51 sutras). Samadhi is a state of direct and reliable perception (pramāṇa) where "the seer" (Purusha, pure consciousness, the Self) abides in itself. Samadhi is the main technique the yogi learns by which to calm the workings of the mind, whereafter **Kaivalya**, the isolation of 'the seer' from the impurities of the mind, is attained. The author describes yoga and then the nature and the means of attaining samādhi.

The second verse of this chapter contains the famous definitional verse.
Yogaś citta-vritti-nirodhaḥ"

("Yoga is the cessation of the modification of mind")

This is the classic definition of Yoga and is applicable to all paradigms. Our mind remains in a constant state of turmoil because of an incessant stream of thoughts that cross it, stays for a while, and disappear. It reappears again in a different form. Flow of thoughts thus continues unabated. Majority of these thoughts taking various forms of Vrittis do not stay there for long, nor leave any impact. Often there is no visible coherence in them, but they effectively prevent our mind from reaching a state of concentration.

Acquiring a perfect state of stillness of mind and reaching a stage of thoughtless consciousness is the aim of Raja Yoga. When mind is still, you can see your real self. It is like a pond where the water is calm and still, you can see its bottom clearly. Muddy pond like a mind full of Vrittis prevents you from seeing anything with clarity.

Monks in the Himalayas often give comparative example of a river and its appearance during the rainy season and winters. Heavy rains in the higher reaches of Himalayas bring in lot of mud, tree branches and the river flow in torrents. It is impossible to go across. Any attempt by a passer-by to cross the river will take him along with the flow and may cause serious damage to him. It may even drown him.

During winters, water is clear, cold and runs slowly and smoothly. You can drop a coin and it will be visible. Stand next to it and you can see your image as clearly as you would see in a mirror.

When the mind is stilled, the seer or real Self is revealed:

Tada drishtu swarupeawasthanam.

Then the Seer is established in his own essential, unmodified, and fundamental nature. As soon as the waves have stopped and the water is stilled, we see its bottom.

Vritti sarupyamitrtatra

In other states (other than that of concentration) the Seer is identified with the modifications (of the mind).

While the four aphorisms mentioned above, emphasise on the stillness of mind free of all modifications, Patanjali gives certain pointers towards realization of truth. The fundamental quest of humanity, right since the beginning of the universe is to know the truth.

Satya ki Khoj (Discovery of truth) is the primary mover of our existence. We must know, understand, and realise the truth about all our endeavours. This is essential for the forward evolutionary journey of the entire mankind, and to live a life that is happy, productive, and fulfilling. Science tells us about the behaviour of nature, Medicine tells us about the human physiology and ways of treating disease, illness and means to cure them. These are the disciplines that affect us all. We must know the truth. All inventions, discoveries, technological advances are based upon the knowledge of the truth. Absence of the knowledge of truth gets everyone in trouble and all progress comes to a halt.

Verse 7 gives the pointers.

Pratyaksha anumana aagmaa pramaanani

It says-Direct perception, inference and competent evidence are proofs.

There are three sources of proofs. Pratyaksha, direct perception; whatever we see and feel, is proof if there is nothing to delude the senses. However, when two of our perceptions do not contradict each other, we call it proof, but if any sensory experience is contradicted by the perception received earlier, we do not believe it and need further corroboration.

Secondly, Anumana, inference; We see a sign and from there we draw our own conclusions using circumstantial evidence. For example, a small wet patch in a limited area is not a proof that it has rained, but if a very large area all around shows the presence of water, it is safe to infer that it has rained. All judicial systems the world over, heavily depend upon this paradigm. Very often in a dispute or in commission of crime, direct evidence or an eyewitness is not available. The judge must piece together the available evidence and draw inference from the circumstantial evidence to reach the truth.

Thirdly, Aptavakya, the direct evidence of the experienced and the enlightened ones. The universe is a continuum with many people gaining experience and understanding reality. Their words are proof if they have a reputation of unimpeachable integrity. Truth subsumes knowledge and the knowledgeable ones must be trusted for they bring experience and knowledge that has been tested overtime. A Guru, a teacher, parents fall in that category, whose words are taken as gospel truth. It must be added that trust and faith are essential conditions to gain knowledge. Bhagwat Gita unambiguously emphasises the importance of trust in acquiring any kind of knowledge.

श्रद्धावान् लभते ज्ञानं तत्परः संयतेन्द्रियः |
ज्ञानं लब्ध्वा परां शान्तिमचिरेणाधिगच्छति || 39||CH 4

śhraddhāvānllabhate jñānaṁ tat-paraḥ sanyatendriyaḥ
jñānaṁ labdhvā parāṁ śhāntim achireṇādhigachchhati

śhraddhāvān—a faithful person; labhate—achieves; jñānam—divine knowledge; tat-paraḥ—devoted (to that); sanyata—controlled; indriyaḥ—senses; jñānam—transcendental knowledge; labdhvā—having achieved; parām—supreme; śhāntim—peace; achireṇa—without delay; adhigachchhati—attains

Those whose faith is deep and who have practiced controlling their mind and senses attain divine knowledge. Through such transcendental knowledge, they quickly attain everlasting supreme peace.

Krishna now introduces the concept of faith in the context of knowledge. Not all spiritual truths are immediately perceptible; some of them can only be experienced after having attained sufficient elevation on the path. If we only accept what we can presently verify or comprehend, we will be bereft of the higher spiritual secrets. Faith helps us accept what we cannot understand at present.

guru vedānta vākyeṣhu dṛiḍho viśhvāsaḥ śhraddhā [v37]

"Faith means firm confidence in the words of the Guru and the scriptures." When such faith is placed upon a wrong personality, it can lead to disastrous consequences. But when it is placed on the true Guru, it opens the pathway for eternal good and welfare.

However, blind faith is not a desirable thing. Before placing it on any Guru, we must use our intellect to confirm that the Guru has realized the Absolute Truth, and he is teaching it in accordance with the eternal Vedic scriptures. Once this is confirmed, then we should strive to deepen our faith in such a Guru and surrender to God under his guidance. The Shvetashvatar Upaniṣhad states:

yasya deve parā bhaktir yathā deve tathā gurau
tasyaite kathitā hyarthāḥ prakāśhante mahātmanaḥ
(6.23) [v38]

"The imports of all the Vedic knowledge are revealed within the hearts of those who engage with unflinching faith in devotion toward Guru and God."

The principles and practice of Raja Yoga are primarily designed to calm the mind through meditation. Our mind is in a state of constant turmoil and must be stilled to get a clear understanding of the Self. Verses 33 to 40 describe in detail seven practices to achieve this state. There is a brief description to understand and follow them.

33. Our Chitta can be pacified if we show Friendship, mercy, gladness, and indifference towards the subjects that are happy, unhappy, good or evil respectively.

34. By throwing out and restraining the Breath.

35. Forms of concentration that bring extraordinary sense-perceptions help build perseverance in our mind.

36. Meditating on the Self Effulgent Light which is beyond all sorrow strengthens concentration.

37. Meditating on the heart that has given up all attachment to the sense objects helps in concentration.

38. Meditating on the knowledge that one experiences during sleep through dreams.

39. Anything that appeals to oneself as good also builds concentration.

40. Meditating thus, one's mind is completely unobstructed from the smallest to the infinite.

These are some of the practices recommended by Patanjali for calming the mind. However, it is essential to prepare oneself by purifying the mind which is subjected to numerous impurities by its contact with the external world, desires and negativity that permeates the eco-system.

Ashtanga Yoga that forms an integral part of Raja Yoga has eight limbs that are mentioned in verse number 29, chapter 2 0f the Yoga Sutra.

First five out of these eight limbs are essentially meant for purification and provide deep insight into the classic format of Yoga. These eight limbs are as follows.

- **Yama**
- **Niyama**
- **Asana**
- **Pranayama**
- **Pratyahara**
- **Dharana**
- **Dhyana**
- **Samadhi**

1. ***Yama*** – restraints or ethics of behaviour; Yama consists of:
Ahimsa (Non-violence)
Satya (Truthfulness)
Asteya (Non stealing)
Brahmacharya (Chastity)
Aparigraha (Non possession)

These are great vows that must be taken by every individual regardless of the time, place, purpose, and caste-rules. Non-violence and truthfulness remove all enmities. By the establishment of non-stealing all wealth comes to a Yogi. By observing continence, considerable energy is gained.

Aparigraha or non-receiving is a great quality and brings purity of heart. Usually, we are beholden to others to receive some gifts or favour. With every gift, you are likely to receive the evils of the giver. If he does not receive, the mind is purified and the first power it gets is memory of past life. Only then the practitioner becomes fixed in his ideal.

2. ***Niyama*** – observances; Niyama consists of:
Saucha (Cleanliness)
Santosha (Contentment)
Tapas (Austerity)
Svadhyaya (Self-study)
Isvara Pranidhana (Devotion to the lord)

External purification is keeping the body pure. A person who does not observe basic hygiene can never be a Yogi. There must be internal purification too. Indeed, internal purity is of greater value than the external, but both are necessary as a condition precedent to the practice of Yoga. There also arises purification of Sattva, cheerfulness of the mind, concentration, conquest of the organs and fitness for the realisation of the self.

To the yogi everything is bliss, every human face that he sees brings cheerfulness to him. That is the sign of a virtuous man. If you are in misery, do not go outside and inflict your misery on others. When your mind is controlled, you have control on your body and it becomes your slave,

It is also essential to fix your mind on God, surrender to Him. Chanting of mantra regularly helps in achieving this state.

By sacrificing all to God comes Samadhi and by resignation to the Lord, Samadhi becomes perfect.

Having observed the tenets of Yama and Niyama, the practitioner now must move to acquire the right posture to perform various **Asanas.** Verse 46 of chapter 2 of Yog sutra says that the posture should be firm and pleasant.

3. Asanas

Posture is that which is firm and pleasant. Out of the eight components of ashtanga Yoga, Asana is the only one which has deep physical implications and deals with the body, its posture and various forms that have been developed by Yoga Gurus to discipline the body so that it is ready to move on to the next level of Dharana and Samadhi. All other seven limbs of Ashtanga Yoga are subtle in nature and relate to our mind.

स्थिर सुखम आसनम *(Yoga Sutra chapter 2 verse 46)*

It is important to get a firm seat that is pleasant and does not cause an distractions, or else it will be difficult to perform breathing and othe exercises essential for taking the practice of Yoga to its logical conclusion Any kind of disturbance in the body will cause disturbance in the nerve and it will become difficult to concentrate the mind.

Further in verse 47 and 48, Patanjali says that by lessening the tendenc for restlessness and meditating on the unlimited, posture becomes firm and pleasant. In that state, the dualities, good or bad, heat or cold, and al pairs of opposites will not then disturb you.

Overtime, several Yoga schools have developed multiple forms o Asanas, and some are customised to suit a person depending upon hi strength and capabilities. Surya Namaskar, Vajra asana, Mayur asana Shava asana and many more forms are taught and practised. However, it i essential that the beginners learn these asanas under the supervision of a experienced and a competent teacher. Wrong postures can lead to certai complications and deformities that may cause life-long problems.

Similar process is explained beautifully in Verses 12 and 13 of Chapter 6 o Bhagwat Gita

तत्रैकाग्रं मनः कृत्वा यतचित्तेन्द्रियक्रियः |
उपविश्यासने युञ्ज्याद्योगमात्मविशुद्धये || 12||CH 6

समं कायशिरोग्रीवं धारयन्नचलं स्थिरः |
सम्प्रेक्ष्य नासिकाग्रं स्वं दिशश्चानवलोकयन् || 13||CH 6

tatraikāgraṁ manaḥ kṛitvā yata-chittendriya-kriyaḥ
upaviśhyāsane yuñjyād yogam ātma-viśhuddhaye
samaṁ kāya-śhiro-grīvaṁ dhārayann achalaṁ sthiraḥ
samprekṣhya nāsikāgraṁ svaṁ diśhaśh chānavalokayan

tatra—there; eka-agram—one-pointed; manaḥ—mind; kṛitvā—having made; yata-chitta—controlling the mind; indriya—senses; kriyaḥ—activities; upaviśhya—being seated; āsane—on the seat; yuñjyāt yogam—should strive to practice yog; ātma viśhuddhaye—for purification of the mind; samam—straight; kāya—body; śhiraḥ—head; grīvam—neck; dhārayan—holding; achalam—unmoving; sthiraḥ—still; samprekṣhya—gazing; nāsika-agram—at the tip of the nose; svam—own; diśhaḥ—directions; cha—and; anavalokayan—not looking

Seated firmly on it, the yogi should strive to purify the mind by focusing it on meditation with one pointed concentration, controlling all thoughts and activities. He must hold the body, neck, and head firmly in a straight line, and gaze at the tip of the nose, without allowing the eyes to wander.

Krishna in chapter 6, verse 16 and 17 recommends complete moderation in our daily habits of eating, sleeping and other engagements relating to work, to be eligible for sound Yoga practice. Those indulging more than any kind are not fit to perform Yoga.

नात्यश्नतस्तु योगोऽस्ति न चैकान्तमनश्नतः |
न चाति स्वप्नशीलस्य जाग्रतो नैव चार्जुन || 16||CH 6

nātyaśhnatastu yogo 'sti na chaikāntam anaśhnataḥ
na chāti-svapna-śhīlasya jāgrato naiva chārjuna

na—not; ati—too much; aśhnatah—one who eats; tu—however; yogah—Yog; asti—there is; na—not; cha—and; ekāntam—at all; anaśhnatah—abstaining from eating; na—not; cha—and; ati—too much; svapna-śhīlasya—one who sleeps; jāgratah—one who does not sleep enough; na—not; eva—certainly; cha—and; arjuna—Arjun

O Arjun, those who eat too much or too little, sleep too much or too little, cannot attain success in Yog.

Commentary

After describing the object of meditation and the end-goal achieved by it, Krishna gives some regulations to follow. He states that those who break the rules of bodily maintenance cannot be successful in Yog. Often beginners on the path, with their incomplete wisdom state: "You are the soul and not this body. So simply engage in spiritual activity, forgetting about the maintenance of the body."

However, such a philosophy cannot get one too far. It is true that we are not the body, yet the body is our carrier as long as we live, and we are obliged to take care of it. The Ayurvedic text, Charak Samhitā states: *śharīra mādhyaṁ khalu dharma sādhanam* [v11]

"The body is the vehicle for engaging in religious activity." If the body becomes unwell, then spiritual pursuits get impeded too.

The Ramayan states: *tanu binu bhajana veda nahiṅ varanā* [v12]

"The Vedas do not recommend that we ignore the body, while engaging in spirituality." In fact, they instruct us to take good care of our body with the help of material science. The Īśhopaniṣhad states:

andhaṁ tamaḥ praviśhanti ye 'vidyām upāsate
tato bhūya iva te tamo ya u vidyāyām ratāḥ (9) [v13]

"Those who cultivate only material science go to hell. But those who cultivate only spiritual science go to an even darker hell." Material science is necessary for the maintenance of our body, while spiritual science is necessary for the manifestation of the internal divinity within us. We must balance both in our lives to reach the goal of life. Hence, *yogāsans*, *prāṇāyām*, and the science of proper diet are an essential part of Vedic knowledge. Each of the four Vedas has its associate Veda for material knowledge. The associate Veda of Atharva Veda is Ayurveda, which is the hoary science of medicine and good health. This demonstrates that the Vedas lay emphasis on the maintenance of physical health. Accordingly, Krishna says that overeating or not eating at all, extreme activity, or complete inactivity, etc. are all impediments to Yog. Spiritual practitioners should take good care of their body, by eating fresh nutritious food, doing daily exercise, and getting the right amount of sleep every night.

युक्ताहारविहारस्य युक्तचेष्टस्य कर्मसु ।
युक्तस्वप्नावबोधस्य योगो भवति दुःखहा || 17||CH 6

yuktāhāra-vihārasya yukta-cheṣhṭasya karmasu
yukta-svapnāvabodhasya yogo bhavati duḥkha-hā

yukta—moderate; āhāra—eating; vihārasya—recreation; yukta cheṣhṭasya karmasu—balanced in work; yukta—regulated; svapna-avabodhasya—sleep and wakefulness; yogah—Yog; bhavati—becomes; duḥkha-hā—the slayer of sorrows

But those who are temperate in eating and recreation, balanced in work, and regulated in sleep, can mitigate all sorrows by practicing Yog.

Commentary

Yoga is the union of the soul with God. The opposite of Yoga is *bhog*, which means engagement in sensual pleasures. Indulgence in *bhog* violates the natural laws of the body, and results in *rog* (disease). As stated in the previous verse, if the body becomes diseased, it impedes the practice of Yog. Thus, in this verse, Krishna states that by being temperate in bodily activities and practicing Yoga, we can become free from the sorrows of the body and mind.

The same instruction was repeated two-and-a-half millennium after Krishna by Gautam Buddha, when he recommended the golden middle path between severe asceticism and sensual indulgence. There is a beautiful story regarding this. It is said that before gaining enlightenment, Gautam Buddha once gave up eating and drinking, and sat in meditation. However, after a few days of practicing in this manner, the lack of nourishment made him weak and dizzy, and he found it impossible to steady his mind in meditation. At that time, some village women happened to be passing by. They were carrying water pots on their heads that they had filled from the river nearby and were singing a song. The words of the song were: "Tighten the strings of the *tānpurā* (a stringed Indian musical instrument, resembling a guitar). But do not tighten them so much that the strings break." Their words entered the ears of Gautam Buddha, and he exclaimed, "These illiterate village women are singing such words of wisdom. They contain a message for us humans. We too should tighten our bodies (practice austerities), but not to the extent that the body is destroyed."

Benjamin Franklin (1706 – 1790), a founding father of the United States, is highly regarded as a self-made man. To build his character, starting at the age of 20, he maintained a diary in which he tracked his performance related to the 13 activities he wanted to grow in. The first activity was "Temperance: Eat not to dullness; drink not to elevation."

4. ***Pranayama*** **– control of the** prana**(breath)**

The fourth limb of Ashtanga Yoga is Pranayama.

Verses 49 to 52 of chapter 2 of Yoga Sutras, describe the essential features of Pranayama. This is available to everyone and can be practised independently of other limbs, albeit with care and caution.

Controlling the motion of exhalation and the inhalation is called Pranayama. When posture has been conquered, then the motion of the Prana is to be broken and controlled. Prana is not breath but constitutes controlling of the vital forces of the body. It verily is the sum of the cosmic energy. It is the energy that is present in everybody, and its most apparent manifestation is the free motion of lungs. This motion is caused by Prana drawing in the breath, and it is what we seek to control in Pranayama. We begin by controlling the breath, as the easiest way of getting control of the Prana.

Its modifications are either external or internal, or motionless, regulated by place, time, and number, either long or short. The three sorts of motion of Pranayama are, one by which we draw the breath in, another by which we throw it out, and the third action is when the breath is held in the lungs or stopped from entering the lungs. These again are varied in by place and time. By place is meant that the Prana is held to some part of the body. By time is meant how long the Prana should be confined to a certain place, and so we are told how many seconds to keep one motion, and how many seconds to keep another.

The fourth is restraining the Prana by reflecting on external or internal object.

This requires long practice accompanied with reflection.

Our Chitta has by its own nature, all knowledge. It is made of Sattva particles, but is covered by Rajas and Tamas particles, and by Pranayama this covering is removed. After this covering is removed, we can concentrate the mind.

5. ***Pratyahara*** – withdrawal of the senses

Verse 54 of Chapter 2 provides a brief description of Pratyahara.

The drawing in of the organs is by their giving up their own objects and taking the form of the mind-stuff, as it were.

The organs are separate states of the mind-stuff. I see a book; the form is not in the book; it is in the mind. Something is outside which calls that form up. The real form is in the Chitta. The organs identify themselves with, and take the forms of, whatever comes to them. If you can restrain the mind-stuff from taking these forms, the mind will remain calm. This is called Pratyahara.

This process then ensures complete control of the organs.

When a Yogi has succeeded in preventing the organs from taking the forms of external objects, and in making them one with the mind-stuff, then perfect control of organs is achieved. When the organs are perfectly in control, every muscle and nerve will be under control, because the organs are the centres of all sensations, and of all actions. These organs are divided into organs of work and organs of sensation. When the organs are controlled, the Yogi can control all feelings and doings. The whole of the body comes under his control. Then alone one begins to feel joy in being born. When that control of the organs is obtained, we feel how wonderful this body really is. Giving the example of tortoise, similar statement is made by Krishna in Chapter 2, verse 58.

यदा संहरते चायं कूर्मोऽङ्गानीव सर्वशः |
इन्द्रियाणीन्द्रियार्थेभ्यस्तस्य प्रज्ञा प्रतिष्ठिता || 58|| CH 2

yadā sanharate chāyaṁ kūrmo 'ṅgānīva sarvaśhaḥ
indriyāṇīndriyārthebhyas tasya prajñā pratiṣhṭhitā

yadā—when; sanharate—withdraw; cha—and; ayam—this; kūrmaḥ—tortoise; aṅgāni—limbs; iva—as; sarvaśhaḥ—fully; indriyāṇi—senses; indriya-arthebhyaḥ—from the sense objects; tasya—his; prajñā—divine wisdom; pratiṣhṭhitā—fixed in

Translation

When the yogi, like the tortoise drawing back its limbs into its own shell, withdraws all the senses from the sense objects, his wisdom is firmly fixed.

For self-realisation (Moksha) control of the senses is essential. When the senses are drawn back from contact with the sense – objects like sound, colour, etc., then the intellect is rooted in Atma. The same truth is stated by Patanjali in the sutras *Yogaschittavrittinirodhah, tadadrashtuh svarupe Avasthanum.* These two sutras are affirmed by the verse. It means that the senses, which by their nature run after worldly objects should be drawn back, and the mind should be centred in Atma. When this is done firmly, and when there is no deviation from the Self, one's knowledge becomes perfect.

This idea is very clearly brought out by means of an illustration. The tortoise withdraws all its limbs into its own shell at the slightest apprehension of danger from outside. Even if the shell is hacked to pieces it would not extend its limbs. The yogi, like the tortoise, should drawback his senses from the objective world, and settle himself in the Self. It is not enough to restrain one of the senses from one set of objects. Of course, if one sense is controlled, it will make the control of the others easy.

The yogi should withdraw all the senses from all the worldly objects. That is why the word *sarvasah* is used. Even if all the doors are closed except one, through that one door dacoits may enter the house. Even if one window is kept open, a gust of wind from it may extinguish the lamp. So, it is necessary that all the senses should be turned back, and there should be no contact with the external world. It is the sense-organs that make the person aware of the outside world. When they are drawn back there is no external world. In deep sleep, there is no external world because the senses are not functioning. Similarly, the yogi should stop the operation of the senses in his fully conscious state, and then the mind sees the Self within. Sense-restraint is thus the first and foremost of all spiritual disciplines.

When a person learns to control or withdraw the senses from sense objects, as a tortoise retracts its limbs inside its shell in time of danger and cannot be forced to extend its limbs again until the trouble is over, the lamp of Self-knowledge becomes lighted, and one perceives the self-effulgent Supreme Being within. A Self-realized person enjoys the beauty of the world, keeping the senses under complete control like a tortoise. The best way to purify the senses and control them perfectly like a tortoise, is to always engage them in the service of God.

Swami Vivekananda Says —

"As the tortoise can draw in his legs, and if you strike him, not one foot comes out, even so the sage can draw all his sense-organs inside," and nothing can force them out. Nothing can shake him, no temptation or anything. Let the universe tumble about him, it does not make one single ripple in his mind.

As the tortoise tucks its feet and head inside the shell, and you may kill it and break it in pieces, and yet it will not come out, even so the character of that man who has control over his motives and organs is unchangeably established. He controls his own inner forces, and nothing can draw them out against his will. By this continuous reflex of good thoughts, good impressions moving over the surface of the mind, the tendency for doing good becomes strong, and as the result we feel able to control the indriyas (the sense-organs, the nerve-centres).

Pratyahara by bringing in complete control of all sense organs, leads a person to a state of स्थितप्रज्ञ (Stable intellect &Stable wisdom). To a question by Arjuna on the definition and the process of achieving that state, Krishna deals with these in verses 54 to 57 of Gita.

अर्जुन उवाच।
स्थितप्रज्ञस्य का भाषा समाधिस्थस्य केशव।
स्थितधीः किं प्रभाषेत किमासीत व्रजेत किम् ॥ 54॥CH 2

arjuna uvācha
sthita-prajñasya kā bhāṣhā samādhi-sthasya keśhava
sthita-dhīḥ kiṁ prabhāṣheta kim āsīta vrajeta kim

arjunaḥ uvācha—Arjun said; sthita-prajñasya—one with steady intellect; kā—what; bhāṣhā—talk; samādhi-sthasya—situated in divine consciousness; keśhava—Shree Krishna, killer of the Keshi Demon; sthita-dhīḥ—enlightened person; kim—what; prabhāṣheta—talks; kim—how; āsīta—sits; vrajeta—walks; kim—how

Arjun said: O Keshav, what is the disposition of one who is situated in divine consciousness? How does an enlightened person talk? How does he sit? How does he walk?

Commentary

The designations *sthita prajña* (one with steady intellect) and *samādhi-stha* (situated in trance) apply to enlightened persons. Having heard from Krishna about the state of perfect yog, or *Samādhi*, Arjun asks a natural question. He wishes to know the nature of the mind of a person who is in this state. Additionally, he wishes to know how this divine state of mind manifests in a person's behaviour.

Beginning with this verse, Arjun asks Krishna sixteen sets of questions. In response, Krishna reveals the deepest secrets of *karm yog, jñāna yog, bhakti yog,* austerity, meditation, etc. The sixteen sets of questions asked by Arjun are:

1. "What is the disposition of one who is situated in divine consciousness? (Verse 2.54)
2. "If you consider knowledge superior to fruitive works, then why do you ask me to wage this terrible war?" (Verse 3.1)
3. "Why is a person impelled to commit sinful acts, even unwillingly, as if by force?" (Verse 3.36)
4. "You were born much after Vivasvan. How am I to understand that in the beginning you instructed this science to him?" (Verse 4.4)

5. "You praised the path of renunciation of actions, and again you praised work with devotion. Please tell me decisively which of the two is more beneficial?" (Verse 5.1)
6. "O Krishna, the mind is very restless, turbulent, strong, and obstinate. It appears to me that it is more difficult to control than the wind." (Verse 6.34)
7. "What is the fate of the unsuccessful yogi who begins the path with faith, but whose mind deviates from God due to untamed passions, and is unable to reach the highest perfection in this life?" (Verse 6.37)
8. "What is *Brahman* and what is karma? What is *Adhibhūta*, and who are the *Ādhidaiva*? Who is *Ādhiyajña* and how does he dwell in this body? O slayer of the Madhu demon, how can those of steadfast mind be united with you at the time of death?" (Verse 8.1-2)
9. "Please describe to me your divine opulence, by which you pervade all the worlds." (Verse 10.16)
10. "I long to see your cosmic form, O Supreme divine Personality." (Verse 11.3)
11. "You, who existed before all creation, I wish to know who you are, for your nature and workings mystify me." (Verse 11.31)
12. "Between those who are steadfastly devoted to your personal form and those who worship the formless *Brahman*, whom do you consider to be more perfect in Yog?" (Verse 12.1)
13. "I wish to know about *Prakṛiti* (Nature) and *Puruśh* (the enjoyer). What is the field of activities, and who is the knower of the field? What is the nature of knowledge, and the object of knowledge?" (Verse 13.1)
14. "What are the characteristics of those who have gone beyond the three *guṇas*, O Lord? How do they act? How have they passed beyond the bondage of the *guṇas*?" (Verse 14.21)
15. "Where do they stand who disregard the injunctions of the scriptures, but still worship with faith?" (Verse 17.1
16. "I wish to understand the nature of *sanyās* (renunciation), and how it is distinct from *tyāg*, or renouncing the fruits of actions." (Verse 18.1)

श्रीभगवानुवाच ।
प्रजहाति यदा कामान्सर्वान्पार्थ मनोगतान् ।
आत्मन्येवात्मना तुष्टः स्थितप्रज्ञस्तदोच्यते || 55||CH 2

śhrī bhagavān uvācha
prajahāti yadā kāmān sarvān pārtha mano-gatān
ātmany-evātmanā tuṣhṭaḥ sthita-prajñas tadochyate

śhrī-bhagavān uvācha—The Supreme Lord said; prajahāti—discards; yadā—when; kāmān—selfish desires; sarvān—all; pārtha—Arjun, the son of Pritha; manaḥ-gatān—of the mind; ātmani—of the self; eva—only; ātmanā—by the purified mind; tuṣhṭaḥ—satisfied; sthita-prajñaḥ—one with steady intellect; tadā—at that time; uchyate—is said

Translation

The Supreme Lord said: O Parth, when one discards all selfish desires and cravings of the senses that torment the mind, and becomes satisfied in the realization of the self, such a person is said to be transcendentally situated.

Commentary

Krishna begins answering Arjun's questions here and continues till the end of the chapter. Each fragment is naturally drawn towards its whole; just as a piece of stone is drawn by the force of gravitation towards the earth. The individual soul is a fragment of God, who is infinite bliss. Hence, the soul is a fragment of the ocean of infinite bliss, and it experiences the natural urge for bliss. When it strives to relish the bliss of the soul from God, it is called "Divine Love." But when, in ignorance of its spiritual nature, it thinks of itself as the body, and seeks to relish the bliss of the body from the world, it is called "lust."

This world has been called *mṛiga tṛiṣhṇā* in the scriptures, meaning "like the mirage seen by the deer." The sun rays reflecting on the hot desert sand create an illusion of water for the deer. It thinks there is water ahead of it and runs to quench its thirst. But the more it runs toward the water, the more the mirage fades away. Its dull intellect cannot recognize that it is running after an illusion. The unfortunate deer keeps chasing the illusory water and dies of exhaustion on the desert sand. Similarly, the material energy Maya too creates an illusion of happiness, and we run after that illusory happiness in the hope of quenching the thirst of our senses. But no matter how much we try; happiness keeps fading further away from us. The Garuḍ Purāṇ states:

chakradharo 'pi suratvaṁ suratvalābhe sakalasurapatitvam
bhavtirum surapatirūrdhvagatitvaṁ tathāpi nanivartate tṛiṣhṇā (2.12.14)
[v47]

"A king wishes to be the emperor of the whole world; the emperor aspires to be a celestial god; a celestial god seeks to be Indra, the king of heaven; and Indra desires to be Brahma, the secondary creator. Yet the thirst for material enjoyment does not get satiated."

But when one learns to turn the mind away from material allurements and renounces the desires of the senses, such a person comes in touch with the inner bliss of the soul and becomes transcendentally situated. The Kaṭhopaniṣhad goes to the extent of saying that one who has renounced desires becomes like God:

yadā sarve pramuchyante kāmā ye 'sya hṛidi śhritaḥ
atha martyo 'mṛito bhavatyatra brahma samaśhnute (2.3.14) [v48]

"When one eliminates all selfish desires from the heart, then the materially fettered *jīvātmā* (soul) attains freedom from birth and death and becomes Godlike in virtue." Krishna states in the above verse that a transcendentally situated person is one who has given up selfish desires and cravings of the senses and is satisfied in the self.

दुःखेष्वनुद्विग्नमनाः सुखेषु विगतस्पृहः ।
वीतरागभयक्रोधः स्थितधीर्मुनिरुच्यते || 56||**CH 2**
duḥkheṣhv-anudvigna-manāḥ sukheṣhu vigata-spṛihaḥ
vīta-rāga-bhaya-krodhaḥ sthita-dhīr munir uchyate

duḥkheṣhu—amidst miseries; anudvigna-manāḥ—one whose mind is undisturbed; sukheṣhu—in pleasure; vigata-spṛihaḥ—without craving; vīta—free from; rāga—attachment; bhaya—fear; krodhaḥ—anger; sthita-dhīḥ—enlightened person; muniḥ—a sage; uchyate—is called

Translation

One whose mind remains undisturbed amidst misery, who does not crave for pleasure, and who is free from attachment, fear, and anger, is called a sage of steady wisdom.

Commentary

In this verse, Krishna describes sages of steady wisdom as: 1) *Vīta rāga*—they give up craving for pleasure, 2) *Vīta bhaya*—they remain free from fear, 3) *Vīta krodha*—they are devoid of anger.

An enlightened person does not allow the mind to harbour the material frailties of lust, anger, greed, envy, etc. Only then can the mind steadily contemplate on transcendence and be fixed in the divine. If one permits the mind to brood over miseries, then the contemplation on the divine ceases and the mind is dragged down from the transcendental level. The process of torture works in the same manner. More than the present pain itself, it is the memories of past pain and apprehensions of future pain that torment the mind. But when the mind drops these two and must simply grope with the present sensation, the pain surprisingly shrinks to a manageable (within the limits of tolerance) size. It is well known that historically Buddhist monks adopted a similar technique for tolerating torture from invading conquerors.

Similarly, if the mind craves external pleasures, it runs to the objects of enjoyment, and is again diverted from divine contemplation. So, a sage of steady wisdom is one who does not allow the mind to hanker for pleasure or lament for miseries. Further, such a sage does not permit the mind to succumb to the urges of fear and anger. In this way, the mind becomes situated on the transcendental level.

यः सर्वत्रानभिस्नेहस्तत्तत्प्राप्य शुभाशुभम् |
नाभिनन्दति न द्वेष्टि तस्य प्रज्ञा प्रतिष्ठिता || 57||z

yaḥ sarvatrānabhisnehas tat tat prāpya śhubhāśhubham
nābhinandati na dveṣhṭi tasya prajñā pratiṣhṭhitā

yaḥ—who; sarvatra—in all conditions; anabhisnehaḥ—unattached; tat—that; tat—that; prāpya—attaining; śhubha—good; aśhubham—evil; na—neither; abhinandati—delight in; na—nor; dveṣhṭi—dejected by; tasya—his; prajñā—knowledge; pratiṣhṭhitā—is fixed

Translation

One who remains unattached under all conditions and is neither delighted by good fortune nor dejected by tribulation, he is a sage with perfect knowledge.

Commentary

Rudyard Kipling, a famous British poet, has encapsulated the essence of this verse on Sthita prajña (Sage of steady intelligence) in his famous poem "If." Here are a few lines from the poem:

If you can dream—and not make dreams your master;
If you can think—and not make thoughts your aim,
If you can meet with Triumph and Disaster
And treat those two impostors just the same…
If neither foes nor loving friends can hurt you,
If all men count with you, but none too much:

If you can fill the unforgiving minute
With sixty seconds' worth of distance run,
Yours is the Earth and everything that's in it,
And—which is more—you'll be a Man, my son!

The popularity of this poem shows the natural urge in people to reach the state of enlightenment, which Krishna describes to Arjun. One may wonder how an English poet expressed the same state of enlightenment that is described by the Supreme Lord. The fact is that the urge for enlightenment is the intrinsic nature of the soul. Hence, knowingly, or unknowingly, everyone craves for it, in all cultures around the world. Krishna is describing it here, in response to Arjun's question.

1.Dharana

Pratyahara and deep practice of all preceding four limbs, Yama, Niyama, Asana, and Pranayama enables the mind to become fit for Dharana.

After all covering has been removed, we are able to concentrate the mind.

Chapter 3 of Yoga Sutras, verse 1 to 4 define the essence of Dharana, Dhyana and Samadhi.

Dharana is holding the mind on to a particular object.

Dharana (Concentration) is when the mind holds on to some object, either in the body, or outside the body, and keeps itself in that state.

An unbroken flow of knowledge in that object is Dhyana. The mind tries to think of one object, to hold itself to one spot, as the top of the head, the heart, etc., and if the mind succeeds in receiving the sensations only through that part of the body, and through no other part, that would be **Dharana.**

When the mind succeeds in keeping itself in that state for some time, it is called **Dhyana** (meditation)

When that, giving up all forms, reflects only the meaning, it is Samadhi.

That comes when in meditation the form or the external part is given up. Suppose I were meditating on a book, and that I have gradually succeeded in concentrating the mind on it, and perceiving only the internal sensations, the meaning, unexpressed in any form-that state of Dhyana is called **Samadhi.**

Dharana, Dhyana and Samadhi when practised regarding one object is described as Samyama. (संयम)

When someone can direct his mind to a particular object and fix it there, and then keep it there for a long time, separating the object from the internal part, this is called Samyama; or Dharana, Dhyana, and Samadhi, one following the other, and making one. The form of the thing has vanished, and only its meaning remains in the mind.

When one has succeeded in making this Samyama, all powers come under his control. This is the great instrument of the yogi. The objects of knowledge are infinite, and they are divided into gross, grosser, grossest and fine, finer, finest, and so on. Samyama should be first applied to gross things, and when you begin to get knowledge of the gross, slowly, by stages, it should be applied to finer things. This should be applied in stages and not attempt to go too fast.

By the suppression of the disturbed impressions of the mind, and by the rise of impressions of control, the mind, which persists in that moment of control, is said to attain the controlling modifications.

The flow of this continuous control of the mind becomes steady when practised day after day, and the mind obtains the faculty of constant concentration.

It is possible to evaluate the situation when the mind has become concentrated. In this state the idea of time will vanish. The more time passes unnoticed the more concentrated we are. In our routine life we see that when we are interested in a book, we do not note the time at all; and when we leave the book, we are often surprised to find how many hours have passed. All time will have the tendency to come and stand in the one present. We can define the state of concentration.

"When the past and present come and stand in one, the mind is said to be concentrated".

Verse 56 of chapter 3 of Yoga Sutra describes the highest state that a person can achieve through the practice of Raja Yoga-Kaivalya. It says that by the similarity of purity between the Sattva and the Purusha comes Kaivalya.

When the soul realises that it depends on nothing in the universe, from gods to the lowest atom, that is called Kaivalya (isolation) and perfection. It is attained when this mixture of purity and impurity called Sattva (intellect) has been made as pure as the Purusha itself; then the sattva reflects only the unqualified essence of purity, which is the Purusha.

Concentration, mindfulness, one-pointedness, absolute focus is synonymous, and they are all designed to create a state of thoughtless consciousness. Concentration is samadhi, and that is Yoga power; That is the principal theme of this science, and it is the highest means. Samadhi is the means through which we can gain anything and everything, mental, moral, or spiritual.

The ancient Chinese philosopher Lao Tzu once stated, "To the mind that is still, the entire universe surrenders." When we allow our minds to be quiet, we begin to see life in a whole new light.

Among all the minds that we see in various disciplines, only that mind that has attained Samadhi, perfect concentration is the highest. A person who has attained certain powers through medicines, or through words, or through mortifications, still has desires, but that person who has attained to samadhi through concentration is alone free from all desires. Desires are indeed the biggest impediment to liberation-the highest goal of mankind.

Yogi does not perceive any work as black nor white; for others they are threefold-black, white, and mixed. When the yogi has attained perfection, his actions, and the Karmas produced by those actions, do not bind him, because he did not desire them. He just works on; he works to do good, and he does good, but does not care for the results, and it will not come to him. But for the ordinary men, who have not attained to the highest state, works are of three kinds, black (evil actions), white (good actions), and mixed.

A yogi performs all works that come to him, but he performs them as offerings to God and does not do them for the sake of the result. He then is not bound by the Karmic circle. Krishna in chapter 3 verse 9-.

यज्ञार्थात्कर्मणोऽन्यत्र लोकोऽयं कर्मबन्धनः |
तदर्थं कर्म कौन्तेय मुक्तसङ्गः समाचर || 9||CH 3

yajñārthāt karmaṇo 'nyatra loko 'yaṁ karma-bandhanaḥ
tad-arthaṁ karma kaunteya mukta-saṅgaḥ samāchara

yajña-arthāt—for the sake of sacrifice; karmaṇaḥ—than action; anyatra—else; lokaḥ—material world; ayam—this; karma-bandhanaḥ—bondage through one's work; tat—that; artham—for the sake of; karma—action; kaunteya—Arjun, the son of Kunti; mukta-saṅgaḥ—free from attachment; samāchara—perform properly

Work must be done as a yajna to the Supreme Lord; otherwise, work causes bondage in this material world. Therefore, O son of Kunti, for the satisfaction of God, perform your prescribed duties, without being attached to the results.

Commentary

A knife in the hands of a robber is a weapon for intimidation or committing murder, but in the hands of a surgeon is an invaluable instrument used for saving people's lives. The knife is neither murderous nor benedictory—its effect is determined by how it is used. As Shakespeare said: "For there is nothing good or bad, but thinking makes it so." Similarly, work is neither good nor bad. Depending upon the state of the mind, it can be either binding or elevating. Work done for the enjoyment of one's senses and the gratification of one's pride is the cause of bondage in the material world, while work performed as *yajna* (sacrifice) for the pleasure of the Supreme Lord liberates one from the bonds of Maya and attracts divine grace. Since it is our nature to perform actions, we are forced to work in one of the two modes. We cannot remain without working for even a moment as our mind cannot remain still.

If we do not perform actions as a sacrifice to God, we will be forced to work to gratify our mind and senses. Instead, when we perform work as a sacrifice, we then look upon the whole world and everything in it as belonging to God, and therefore, meant for utilization in his service. A beautiful ideal for this was established by King Raghu, the ancestor of Lord Ram. Raghu performed the *Vishwajeet* sacrifice, which requires donating all of one's possessions in charity.

sa viśhwajitam ājahre yajñaṁ sarvasva dakṣhiṇam
ādānaṁ hi visargāya satāṁ vārimuchām iva (Raghuvanśh 4.86) [v5]

"Raghu performed the *Vishwajeet yajna* with the thought that just as clouds gather water from the Earth, not for their enjoyment, but to shower it back upon the Earth, similarly, all he possessed as a king had been gathered from the public in taxes, not for his pleasure, but for the pleasure of God. So, he decided to use his wealth to please God by serving his citizens with it." After the *yajna*,

Raghu donated all his possessions to his citizens. Then, donning the rags of a beggar and holding an earthen pot, he went out to beg for his meal.

While resting under a tree, he heard a group of people discussing, "Our king is so benevolent. He has given away everything in charity." Raghu was pained on hearing his praise and spoke out, "What are you discussing?" They answered, "We are praising our king. There is nobody in the world as charitable as him." Raghu retorted, "Do not ever say that again. Raghu has given nothing." They said, "What kind of person are you who are criticizing our king? Everyone knows that Raghu has donated everything he owned." Raghu replied, "Go and ask your king that when he came into this world, did he possess anything? He was born empty-handed, is it not? Then what was his that he has given away?"

This is the spirit of *Karm Yog*, in which we see the whole world as belonging to God, and hence meant for the satisfaction of God. We then perform our duties not for gratifying our mind and senses, but for the pleasure of God. Lord Vishnu instructed the Prachetas in this fashion:

gṛiheṣhv āviśhatāṁ chāpi puṁsāṁ kuśhala-karmaṇām
mad-vārtā-yāta-yāmānāṁ na bandhāya gṛihā matāḥ (Bhāgavatam 4.30.19)
[v6]

"The perfect *Karm yogis*, even while fulfilling their household duties, perform all their works as *yajna* to me, knowing me to be the Enjoyer of all activities. They spend whatever free time they have in hearing and chanting my glories. Such people, though living in the world, never get bound by their actions."

We often feel dissatisfied by the kind of work we are required to perform, even though it is consistent with our inherent nature and tend to abandon it. This often happens on account of how others perceive that work, and we get influenced by their opinion. Krishna advises against it in the following verse from chapter 18.

सहजं कर्म कौन्तेय सदोषमपि न त्यजेत् ।
सर्वारम्भा हि दोषेण धूमेनाग्निरिवावृता: || 48||CH 18

saha-jaṁ karma kaunteya sa-doṣham api na tyajet
sarvārambhā hi doṣheṇa dhūmenāgnir ivāvṛitāḥ

saha-jam—born of one's nature; karma—duty; kaunteya—Arjun, the son of Kunti; sa-doṣham—with defects; api—even if; na tyajet—one should not abandon; sarva-ārambhāḥ—all endeavors; hi—indeed; doṣhena—with evil; dhūmena—with smoke; agniḥ—fire; iva—as; āvṛitāḥ—veiled

One should not abandon duties born of one's nature, even if one sees defects in them, O son of Kunti. Indeed, all endeavours are veiled by some evil, as fire is by smoke.

Commentary

People sometimes recoil from their duty because they see a defect in it. Here, Krishna states that no work is free from defect, just as fire naturally has smoke on top of it. For example, we cannot breathe without killing millions of microbes. If we cultivate the land, we destroy innumerable microorganisms. If we succeed against competition in business, we deprive others of wealth. When we eat, we deprive another of food. Since *swa-dharma* entails activity, it cannot be devoid of defects.

But the benefits of the *swa-dharma* far outweigh its defects. And the foremost benefit is that it provides a comfortable and natural path for one's purification and elevation. In his book, "Making a Life, making a Living), Mark Albion, who was a professor at the Harvard Business School, cites a study in which the careers of 1,500 business school graduates were tracked from 1960 to 1980. From the beginning, graduates were grouped in two categories. In category A were those who said they wanted to make money first, so that they could do what they really wanted to do later, after they had taken care of their financial concerns. Eighty-three percent fell in category A. In category B were those who pursued their interests first, sure that money would eventually follow. Seventeen percent came in category B. After 20 years, there were 101 millionaires. One person was from category A (who wanted to make money first), and one hundred from category B (who pursued their interest first). The overwhelming majority of the people who became wealthy did so thanks to the work they found profoundly absorbing. Mark Albion concludes that for most people there is a difference between work and play. But if they do what they love, then work becomes play, and they never have to work for another day in their life. That is what Krishna is asking Arjun to do—not to abandon the work that is best suited to his nature, even if it has defects in it, rather to work according to his natural propensity. *But for work to be elevating, it must be done in the proper consciousness, described in the next verse.*

असक्तबुद्धिः सर्वत्र जितात्मा विगतस्पृहः |
नैष्कर्म्यसिद्धिं परमां सन्न्यासेनाधिगच्छति || 49||CH 18

asakta-buddhiḥ sarvatra jitātmā vigata-spṛihaḥ
naiṣhkarmya-siddhiṁ paramāṁ sannyāsenādhigachchhati

asakta-buddhiḥ—those whose intellect is unattached; sarvatra—everywhere; jita-ātmā—who have mastered their mind; vigata-spṛihaḥ—free from desires; naiṣhkarmya-siddhim—state of actionlessness; paramām—highest; sanyāsena—by the practice of renunciation; adhigachchhati—attain

Those whose intellect is unattached everywhere, who have mastered the mind, and are free from desires by the practice of renunciation, attain the highest perfection of freedom from action.

Commentary

In this last chapter, Krishna repeats many of the principles he has already explained. In the beginning of this chapter, he explained to Arjun that merely running away from the responsibilities of life is not *sanyās*, nor is it renunciation. Now he describes the state of actionlessness, or *naiṣhkarmya-siddhi*. This state can be reached even amidst the flow of the world by detaching ourselves from events and outcomes, and simply focusing on doing our duty. This is just as water flowing under a bridge enters from one side and flows out from the other. The bridge is neither the recipient of the water nor its distributor; it remains unaffected by its flow. Likewise, the *karm yogis* do their duty, but keep the mind unaffected by the stream of events. They do not neglect putting in their best efforts in doing their duty, as an act of worship to God, but they leave the outcome in his hands, and are thus contented and undisturbed with whatever happens.

Here's a simple story to illustrate this point. A man had two daughters; the first was married to a farmer and the second was married to a brick kiln owner. One day, the father rang up the first daughter and inquired how she was doing. She replied, "Father, we are going through economic hardships. Please pray to God for us that we may have plentiful rains in the coming months." He then rang up the second daughter, and she requested, "Father, we are low on funds. Please request God not to send rains this year, so that we may have lots of sunshine and a good production of bricks." The father heard the opposite requests of his daughters, and thought, "God alone knows what is best. Let him do what he feels is best." Such acceptance of the will of God brings detachment from outcomes, despite being immersed in the incessant stream of events in the world.

It would be important to reflect on the following statement.

"If you do what you want to do, the result would be in the hands of God. If you do what He wants you to do, the result would be in your hands". It is evident that if you act in accordance with the wishes of God, He will help you to achieve what you wish to achieve.

Practice of Raja Yoga calms the mind, indeed helps to master the mind and one can attain perfection in whatever one does without being bound by it. You are no longer subservient to the vanities or the fickle behaviour of the mind which is inherently unstable. To a question by Arjuna about the vagaries and the wavering nature of the mind Krishna counsels him how to control it.

श्रीभगवानुवाच |
असंशयं महाबाहो मनो दुर्निग्रहं चलम् |
अभ्यासेन तु कौन्तेय वैराग्येण च गृह्यते || 35 ||CH 6

śhrī bhagavān uvācha
asanśhayaṁ mahā-bāho mano durnigrahaṁ chalam
abhyāsena tu kaunteya vairāgyeṇa cha gṛihyate

śhrī-bhagavān uvācha—Krishna said, asanśhayam—undoubtedly; mahā-bāho—mighty-armed one; manaḥ—the mind; durnigraham—difficult to restrain; chalam—restless; abhyāsena—by practice; tu—but; kaunteya—Arjun, the son of Kunti; vairāgyeṇa—by detachment; cha—and; gṛihyate—can be controlled

Translation

Doubtless, O mighty Arjuna, the mind is restless and hard to control; but by practice and by detachment, O son of Kunti, it can be restrained.

Commentary

Krishna tells Arjuna that the task of restraining the mind is very difficult because of its restless nature. But there is no need to despair. It can be controlled by practice and dispassion. The great teachers point out that there are ways and means of overcoming the difficulties in the control of the mind. Krishna while admitting the mind's restlessness, speaks about the way to control it, and the way is practice and dispassion.

1. practice (abhyasa), and 2. dispassion(vairagya).

In the world everything causes fear, and in dispassion alone is fearlessness. When dispassion develops, the mind immediately stops thinking of the external world and is immediately drawn into the Self. The joy of vairagya is real, unobstructed, and perennial because it is the joy of the Self, pure and uncontaminated.

Practice (Abhyasa) is the keynote of the Krishna's message for all spiritual aspirants. The baby learns to walk by practice, the child learns to read and write by practice, the architect, the painter, the poet, the musician, the sportsman, the athlete-men of all professions acquire perfection by practice. Where the practice is less, the achievement is also less. Idleness wins nothing, and on the spiritual path idleness is the greatest enemy. All worldly gains have been acquired by hard work and constant application. The man who feels shy of labour remains where he is. Men of ordinary talents have risen in life by systematic practice in their professions of skill.

Dispassion aids spiritual sadhana, and practice aids to strengthen dispassion. The body and the mind function by habit. If the habits are bad, man ruins himself if the habits are good, man saves himself. So, one should practise and develop good habits. If a man is accustomed to visit a wine bar at a particular time in the day, at that exact hour, the body and mind run for the bottle, and nothing can stop him. In the same way, if a man practises meditation at a particular time for a particular period, the body and mind run for it, and nothing can stop him. It is practice. When it is performed systematically and regularly, it becomes automatic, and afterward, no effort is needed to coax the mind and body to do it. As meditation becomes deeper and deeper, the joy felt at that time is so precious that one does not care to think of anything else. He is fully absorbed in it.

The practice, and regular practice is the key to it.

Practice and sense of detachment will certainly help, but in the beginning, mind will waver, used as it is to the distractions caused by multiple material attractions and thoughts. It will not be easy, but there is no short cut to immortality. Here, Krishna knowing the tendencies of our mind, advises the practitioner to bring back the focus on God, or the subject of his concentration whenever the mind wanders away. This will continue to happen and calls for strong will and perseverance.

यतो यतो निश्चरति मनश्चञ्चलमस्थिरम् |
ततस्ततो नियम्यैतदात्मन्येव वशं नयेत् || 26 || CH 6

yato yato niśhcharati manaśh chañchalam asthiram
tatas tato niyamyaitad ātmanyeva vaśhaṁ nayet

yataḥ yataḥ—whenever and wherever; niśhcharati—wanders; manaḥ—the mind; chañchalam—restless; asthiram—unsteady; tataḥ tataḥ—from there; niyamya—having restrained; etat—this; ātmani—on God; eva—certainly; vaśham—control; nayet—should bring

Whenever and wherever the restless and unsteady mind wanders, one should bring it back and continually focus it on God.

Commentary

Success in meditation is not achieved in a day; the path to perfection is long and arduous. When we sit for meditation with the resolve to focus our mind upon God, we will find that ever so often it wanders off in worldly *saṅkalp* and *vikalp*. It is thus important to understand the three steps involved in the process of meditation:

With the intellect's power of discrimination, we decide that the world is not our goal. Hence, we forcefully remove the mind from the world. This requires effort.

Again, with the power of discrimination we understand that God alone is ours, and God-realization is our goal. Hence, we bring the mind to focus upon God. This also requires effort.

The mind comes away from God and wanders back into the world. This does not require effort, it happens automatically.

When the third step happens by itself, *Sadhak's* often become disappointed, "I tried so hard to focus upon God, but the mind went back into the world." Krishna asks us not to feel disappointed. He says the mind is fickle and we should be prepared that it will wander off in the direction of worldly attractions, despite our best efforts to control it. However, when it does wander off, we should once again repeat steps 1 and 2—take the mind away from the world and bring it back to God. Once again, we will experience that step 3 takes place by itself. We should not lose heart, and again repeat steps 1 and 2.

We will have to do this repeatedly. Then slowly, the mind's attachment toward God will start increasing. And simultaneously, its detachment from the world will also increase. As this happens, it will become easier to meditate. But in the beginning, we must be prepared for the battle involved in disciplining the mind. Perseverance is the key.

While different limbs of Ashtanga Yoga have been discussed in detail, a structured protocol needs to be followed to get maximum benefits from this science. In the following paragraphs we will delineate some of these practices to make the experience of meditation real and its consequent benefits.

Practice (Abhyasa) अभ्यास

It is essential to believe that through meditation, which is the uninterrupted flow of the same thought of God, one can easily attain the Highest, for the mind eventually succumbs to a thought to which it is subjected uninterruptedly for a long time. If we continue to imbue the mind with a certain kind of consciousness—whatever may be the condition of the mind in the beginning, whether spiritual or not, whether filled with love for God or with restless desires—in course of time the desired change will take place.

Sri Ramakrishna laid much stress on this fact. It takes time to comprehend his teachings on this subject, but once we understand them, they hold great promise and assurance therein. He used to say that the mind is like a laundered cloth which takes the colour of the dye in which it is dipped. At first, one is inclined to believe that the mind must be made pure before it is plunged into the thought of God to take His colour. There was nothing particularly encouraging in this because the great problem of almost all spiritual aspirants is the attainment of purity of mind. Such purification is three-fourths of the battle; for when it is fully accomplished, spiritual realization comes spontaneously. But as one ponders over Sri Ramakrishna's simile, one begins to understand it differently. In likening the mind to a laundered cloth, he spoke of the average mind, the mind which is so crowded with worldly and contradictory thoughts and feelings, and which is so averse to the thought of God. It was not the purified mind that he likened to a laundered cloth, but the mind in whatever condition it may be. He meant that even this average mind, if dipped in the thought of God, would take on spiritual colour.

Here is a psychological truth, wonderfully encouraging and helpful but often forgotten by spiritual aspirants. Once a man came to Sri Ramakrishna, saying, "I cannot control my mind—I don't know how." The Master, astonished, said, "Why do you not practise abhyasa-yoga?" Bringing the mind back again and again to the thought of God—that is what abhyasa-yoga means. This practice is particularly commended in the Bhagavad Gita. Does it matter very much if the mind wanders in the beginning, so long as you bring it back to Him? If we could remember this, half the battle would be already won, but unfortunately, we often do not, and then we think of other things and completely forget the spiritual quest. Such being the case, it would be useful to discuss certain points concerned with the means of self-control and meditation.

Calmness of mind (Shant Chitta) शांतचित्त

What is the condition of mind suitable for meditation? It is known to all of us, as quietness. This is not a forced calmness, but a calmness resulting from the cessation of most of the strong desires. The things which disturb the mind, whether rising from within or coming from without, relate to our secret, basic desires. We are always trying to realize certain ends. Though we strive desperately, we often fail, and failure exasperates the mind. Even when success is ours, there are strange results. Because the objects of our desires sometimes elude us while we are enjoying them, we feel disappointed and cheated; and when we are not thus frustrated, we become attached to the objects of enjoyment, in which case, since enjoyment cannot be continually intensified, satiety follows. All these reactions keep the mind continually restless, whether in a pleasant or unpleasant mode. Thus, we find that the thoughts which do not allow our mind to dwell on the Presence of God relate to the objects of our desires; and only when we succeed in ridding ourselves of our predominant desires does the mind become comparatively quiet.

We call this state of relative calmness the beginning of pratyahara (withdrawal of the mind), a condition in which the mind, though sometimes restless, is at other times quiet - restless when it meets the objects of desire, but quiet when it does not do so. This is a very favourable state. If you find that your mind is naturally quiet when you are not in actual contact with disturbing things, that you like to be alone and that you have a feeling of serenity, recognize this condition as most desirable. In this condition you should try your best to practise meditation; never neglect it.

We are fully aware that the mind is a very changeable entity. Do not think that any desired condition will continue to exist simply because you have once reached it. Something may arise from within or come from without to distract you, and it may sometimes take five or even ten years for the mind to quiet down again, just as the sea takes days to regain calmness after a storm. It does not mean that we shall never be safe. Undoubtedly there is a mental condition in which one need have no fear at all, but that is an exalted state. When a person has reached that one-pointed state he has burned his bridges behind him: he has reached a condition in which the things of this world can no longer attract him; his mind will never hark back to the world he has left behind. He is secure.

Suppose we have reached the state in which the mind, though at times restless, is at other times quiet. What shall we do then if we want to succeed in meditation? We must at the beginning make a firm resolution to be very regular in our practice. Whatever may be going on, we always manage to attend to our urgent bodily needs; we should be equally faithful to the practice of meditation. Meditation should be as much part of life as breathing. When a person is very busy, he says, "I have no time to breathe." He does not stop breathing. So it should be with meditation, though at first the desire to practise it may appear artificial. Make up your mind; say to yourself, "I must meditate."

We are familiar of a song about a man who, after spending all his life foolishly, finally realized his mistake and said, "I had time for everything else, O Lord, but I did not have time to think of Thee!" Notice this peculiarity of the human mind: there is a time and a place for everything else in our life, but we do not have even fifteen minutes daily for meditation! If you say, you have no time or energy, do you think it is believable? By making such statements we are deceiving ourselves. Where there's a will there's a way. If you are determined, you can always find time to meditate. It simply means prioritizing your goals and pursuing those that have been identified as such.

Sometimes in meditation the mind behaves wonderfully; it becomes calm and concentrated easily, and you are encouraged. But if at other times it behaves badly, refuses to quiet down, and is restless with all kinds of thoughts, you may be tempted to say, "No use for me to meditate. I try but reach nowhere. Unless you are born with wonderful qualities of mind and in a very advanced state of spiritual development, you are subject, like every other man who has tried to become spiritual to these fluctuations of consciousness. Do not let them discourage you, and do not think you are not fit to meditate when your mind is not sufficiently spiritual. Some have asked, "How can I approach God with a low state of mind?" If you were cold, would you say, "I am cold, so let me get warm before approaching the fire"? Or would you say, "I am cold and therefore the first thing to do is to go to the fire and warm myself"? If you feel yourself lacking in spirituality, that is the time of all times to think of God. Do not let your mind mislead you. The mind can trick you in many ways: sometimes it will tempt directly, and again it will mislead in the very name of religion. This reluctance to meditate because you are "not spiritual enough" is a trick the mind plays on you. Whatever your mental condition, even if your mind be filled with low thoughts, try to think about God. Of course, you may not be able to think about Him or meditate on Him as you would wish, but what does it matter? Keep trying. A vicious horse kicks, rears and attempts to throw the rider, but if the rider manages to stay firmly in the saddle, the horse quietens down, knowing it has found its master. The mind behaves in the same way. It will try to dislodge you, but upon finding that you cannot be shaken off, it will become your slave. That is the secret of the mind, so do not bother about its condition. Make the determination to ride it, and this determination, which implies concentration, is itself a victory.

Fixed time for meditation (निश्चित समय)

Next, you must have a fixed time for meditation. Having chosen this path with determination one should meditate not less than twice a day. If you cannot meditate twice, meditate at least once, either in the morning or in the evening. In India we think there are four auspicious hours for meditation: early morning—at least an hour before sunrise, while it is still dark—is a very good time. Of this, more later. The second auspicious hour is noon. I do not know whether any special advantage can be derived from it in the city, but undoubtedly in villages, especially in a tropical country, all is hushed at this time and nature seems to stand still. It is so hot that even birds are silent and hide themselves among the leaves of the trees. People are quiet—often they rest at that time—and there is a definite lull; many use the noon hour for meditation and worship. The third auspicious time for meditation is early evening. Evening is certainly one of the best times in which to meditate. If you can, you may practise meditation shortly before dinner, but it is not advisable to meditate immediately thereafter, as digestion may be impaired, and your health affected. The fourth hour is midnight when one does feel a certain stillness. Where it is quiet, midnight is wonderfully suitable. As a matter of fact, many believe that midnight is the best of all hours for meditation.

Morning meditation has a certain advantage over evening meditation, in that the mind is quiet when you waken from the night's rest. All the impressions of the preceding day are erased, as if someone had come after school and wiped the blackboard clean. Then too, nature is quiet in the early morning and the city is not yet fully awake and stirring. Consequently, you find it easier to quiet the mind. There is another advantage: by meditating before the day has begun you give a spiritual impetus and direction to your mind. Though it may tend to lose some of the spiritual strength and enthusiasm as the day progresses, these will nevertheless remain for many hours and sustain you through most of the day.

It should be mentioned here that some may find meditation more successful in the evening than in the morning. There are those who 'wake up' gradually as the day advances. In the morning they are only half-awake, but towards evening wide awake with clear, sharp minds behaving wonderfully. Such persons undoubtedly will find evening or night meditation more successful. If you cannot avail yourself of any of these hours which are especially suitable for meditation, you should choose the one most convenient to you and make every effort to stick to it. The observation of regular hours of meditation is very important, because the mind functions according to habit. If it is made to think and feel in a certain way at a given time for many days consecutively, it will spontaneously think and feel in the same way whenever that time arrives. If we meditate on God at a specified hour, whenever that hour approaches, our mind, without any effort on our part, will be filled with the consciousness of God. This is no mean advantage to derive from regularity of practice.

Fixed place for meditation (निश्चित स्थान)

Just as you should have regular hours of meditation, so should you have a fixed place in which to meditate. That is one great advantage of temples and churches. Since such places are used for thinking of God, the very air in them becomes charged with His presence and the feeling of purity. You can experience positive vibrations there. You are uplifted by merely going there. An atmosphere like that of a temple or church can be created even in a corner of your own room, for wherever an intense thought is held uninterruptedly, the place becomes charged with the quality of it, probably because the material atmosphere and surroundings relate to the body, which vibrates in accordance with the thoughts of the mind. If our thoughts are pure, our bodies likewise attain to a purity which may be called a spiritual vibration; and naturally, with such a change in the body, the outside atmosphere is also changed.

Thus, the fixed place where you meditate will become charged with energy; it will be so permeated with a spiritual quality that your mind will be filled with the thought of meditation as soon as you come to that place. It will be quieted as if by a magic touch, and you will be conscious of a palpable presence. What a great advantage! You can indeed perform this seeming miracle through the one practice of keeping apart a certain place consecrated to thoughts of God.

Conquering the enemies within (दमन)

When we measure the strength of the subtle enemies which hide in our minds—the passions, impulses, greed and desires—these devices seem to provide a very frail protection. I admit this. The word 'hide' implies that even the best of us have not completely escaped their influence. It is said that one is not wholly free of them until one has touched the feet of God. Just as in winter the garden is cleared of weeds and old growth but with the first rain of spring the tiny seeds left lying in the earth sprout to cover it with green, even so, many subtle thoughts, impressions and desires lie hidden in our minds, waiting to spring up at the first opportunity. Therefore, we must be very careful. We know that all these negative impulses are in our minds and that they would easily cover our whole consciousness if we did not restrain them. Our problem is to keep a great part of our mind—and by degrees a greater and yet greater part of it—free from the domination of wrong impulses and desires, so that with the mind thus freed we can think only of God. In the meantime, what should we do to conquer our desires and adverse impulses? Sometimes they succumb to direct attack, but a flank attack is usually better. Fighting a state of mind directly to conquer it can do more harm than good, for thereby the mind often becomes more and more entangled. The wiser course is not to allow oneself to dwell on the condition of mind to be eradicated. Remember this psychological fact: the more you dwell on a mental condition, the more it is strengthened.

There is a story of a monk who used to sit under a roadside tree to pray and meditate. A woman of ill repute often passed by, and he would say to her, "You should give up your evil ways and try to be good. If you do not, terrible things will happen to you after death." Every time the monk saw the woman, he admonished her similarly. In course of time, they both died, and the messengers of death came to claim their spirits. It is said that a bright messenger brings a golden chariot to carry a good person to heaven, whereas a dark messenger comes when an evil person dies. It happened that the dark messenger came for the monk and the celestial messenger for the woman. The monk was astonished. "I think there has been a mistake," he said. "No," answered the messenger, "there has been no mistake. All is quite right." "How can that be?" asked the monk. The messenger replied gravely, "Though seeming to meditate, you were all the while thinking of the woman and her evil deeds. Did not your mind dwell continually on evil? But the woman asked God for help, saying, 'Lord, I am weak. Save me!' Did not her mind dwell on God more than yours?' The monk could make no answer. This may be an extreme illustration, but it contains a deep psychological truth. It points to a fundamental fact concerning mental action, a fact that you can utilize in your own struggle for self-conquest. When the mind is allowed to dwell on some undesirable quality, it creates a new impression that is many times stronger than the original one. Further recognition of this quality will only make it stronger and stronger until it may even become a complex. I am not saying that you should not restrain your mind, that you should let it be uncontrolled, or as it is called, 'natural'. Nor do I mean that you should ignore your weaknesses. But truly it is often safer not to grapple with these directly. The better strategy is to train the mind to dwell on a new level. First divert it from the thought of your weakness to some innocent and pleasing subject; then lift it by degrees to a higher consciousness. This method of self-constraint does not repress the mind, but rather lifts it from dangerous associations by substituting desirable for undesirable thoughts.

If at present you have some serious fault that seems almost impossible to eradicate, you must have lent it strength and support by thinking of it and indulging in it. Take away that support, and the fault will become weak and will finally die through lack of nourishment. This may not be easy to do, but with practise you can form the habit, and it is a sure way of making spiritual progress. After starving your undesirable thoughts for some time, you will probably find that, while many of them have died, some have remained. Do not be too concerned. Let them remain, so long as they do not gain strength. Keep them cornered, and eventually they also will die. Bad company is one of the most potent causes of mental conflict and disturbance. It would be very well to mix with all kinds of people if we could remain unaffected by their company, but this rarely happens. I do not know of anyone who can do it. Right contacts and association are therefore very important in spiritual life. If you share the company of impure persons and are in frequent contact with wrong things, you will be unable to keep under control the thoughts you are trying to check; they will grow and will finally overcome your mind completely.

Choose your friends and the people you spend time with, very carefully.

Observe asceticism (वैराग्य)

A certain amount of asceticism is necessary for spiritual progress. This does not mean renunciation but implies a life of austerity. Some of you, not eager to meditate, may say, "We shall leave that for our next life," or "We shall take it up a few years hence." Many think that youth is the time to enjoy life, that it is well enough to practise religion after beginning to grow old. In other words, when the world has turned sour, they will go to church wearing a long face and think they have religion. That is not and cannot be religion. What do we bring to God in such a case? A worn-out body and a worn-out mind, scarred through and through. Do you think He is pleased with these? We do not take worm-eaten fruits or wilted flowers to his Altar, but perfect offerings. In the same way, we should give Him the best of ourselves. The offering of a fresh and pure mind pleases Him most.

Those who think religion is exclusively for the old make a profound mistake. The young especially should try to be spiritual, for if religious life begins early and the practices mentioned are undertaken while the mind is still fresh and pure, then by keeping a close watch over the mind one can keep it unspoiled. Under no circumstances should we allow the mind to become affected by the world. Youth is the propitious time for setting to work. Sri Ramakrishna once said to a young college student: "When a man makes a brick, he puts his trademark on it while it is still soft. Then, when the brick is dried in the sun and baked in the kiln, the mark becomes permanent. Even so, if you can put the imprint of God on your mind while it is soft, that imprint can never be effaced, but will remain forever.

Practise asceticism—the more the better; and this does not mean making a wry face as if you have bitten a sour apple. Practising asceticism should give a pleasure like that of riding a spirited horse. Gain the strength to control the forces of your body and mind so that you are not dominated by them. This asceticism is necessary, for without it, meditation is impossible.

All the things discussed so far are important preliminaries; they should be practised each day of our lives and not merely at the beginning of our spiritual quest. He who practises them rightly can at will withdraw his mind completely, because he has gained tremendous control over it. But until you have been fully established in these practices, many of you may find that during meditation the mind takes some time to reach a state of quietude. This fact should be given careful consideration. If you rush about doing and thinking many things immediately before meditation, what success can you expect?

For some time prior to meditation, you should try to be quiet and to feel that you are unrelated to the world, that you have nothing to do with it. As husband, wife, mother, father, child and so on, you have many duties, and there are a thousand things demanding your attention. When approaching God, do you know what you should do? You should go to Him as though the world had never existed for you. Dwell upon the truth about God as the only entity that is real, and all other relationships false and transient. This would be the right feeling in the hour of meditation.

Meditate on eternity beyond time and space (अनंत)

Approach meditation with the feeling of eternity. Who succeeds best in meditation? He who at the time of meditation can feel completely unrelated. Do you understand what that means? Try to imagine what eternity is. It is beyond time and consequently beyond all phenomena; it is a condition—if we may call it so—in which none of these relative things exist. When seeking to think of the eternal Lord, you are trying for the time being to go beyond all relationships. You must say, "I have no body, no mind. Time and space have disappeared. The whole universe has vanished. God alone is." Then only will the mind have that subtle perception which will enable it to feel God's gracious presence. Thus, before you enter the place of meditation, you must leave everything relative outside.

There must indeed be sometime during the day when you feel unrelated—because to be so is your true nature. Though you seem to be related to people, you know these relationships are impermanent. Your true nature is unrelated, and it is in the unrelated condition that you must enter meditation.

By fulfilling the conditions mentioned above, real, and appreciable spiritual progress can be made. But here it must be stated that all spiritual practices, including meditation, depend upon one thing: a great yearning for Truth. Have you that yearning? You may say, "I do not feel it. What then, is the use of meditation?" But is it impossible to create that feeling? The mind's appetite for God can be stimulated deliberately. When by whatever means, the mind is made to yearn for Him, the feeling is no less real than if it had come spontaneously. If you wait for time to bring a natural longing, it may never come. Since this longing is essential, create it. At first your mind will fluctuate. But do not be discouraged by these unstable moods of the mind, and above all do not let yourself be defeated.

Suppose that you are a boy and that another boy in the neighbourhood always tries to browbeat you. He has no right to do it, and you know him to be a coward. What is the proper course to take?

Will you submit to the bully, thinking that you are naturally weak and that to fight him is useless? No, you will deliberately call up the feeling of manliness within you. You will say to yourself, "I refuse to be bullied by him." The next time you confront him, that feeling may partially decline, but you will nevertheless manage to look him in the eye, and you will eventually be brave enough to challenge him. You will have become manly, and you will say, "This is my true nature; I am really strong!"

Continuous and sustainable Effort (सतत प्रयास)

We are acting similarly at every moment. In acquiring a skill or gaining knowledge in school or college, we succeed by repeated effort. At first, what we are trying to acquire is not natural to us, but once mastered, it appears an essential part of ourselves. This is even more true in spiritual life, and we must exert ourselves accordingly. At first everything seems difficult, and you say, "What actually is my nature? Maybe I am just not religious. Perhaps I am not destined to be spiritual." There were times when I too thought the same. I would consider a certain obstruction too great for me and its removal an impossibility. Then I would remind myself that I was not really the body and mind, but the spirit; that the realization of my spiritual self was my destiny. I knew that if I did not conquer the obstruction then, I was just postponing the task for the future. Why not act at once and finish it? I can truly say, my good fortune lay in holding to this thought. True, I was sometimes tempted to give up the struggle, but then I would think, "I cannot escape my spiritual destiny. Let me therefore realize it now!"

Great longing and faith are very important in the practice of meditation, for without intense desire for God and faith in Him, meditation proves half-hearted and sterile. Where there is no interest in what you are doing, it becomes a mere formality, and effort is soon abandoned.

Create an image of a Personal God (ईष्टदेव)

If you believe in a personal God, pray to Him. By 'personal God' I do not mean God with a body, but God with self-consciousness, who is our Father, Mother, Friend, and Lord, who is the all-pervading Creator of the universe. He listens when we pray to Him; we can approach Him in full confidence, just as children approach their parents. Believing in a personal God and loving Him will make it very easy for you to meditate. Dwell on the thought of Him more and more. Do things for Him. Success in spiritual life lies in concentrating every thought, every feeling, every ounce of energy on God.

How will you do it? When you speak, speak of God. When you walk, go to His temple. When you work with your hands, do something in His service. Every function of body and mind must somehow be directed towards Him. If you must go to an office instead of a temple, make your office the temple of God! If your work is honest, it can be done. If it is dishonest, change that work. If changing means even facing starvation, then face it! Courage - that is always necessary. Do not forget this: he who created the world is still behind it and will never let us starve. If we really want the Truth and hence are willing to discard whatever is wrong and untrue, we shall never lose by following the Truth. It is not that things will happen just as we wish, but they will happen with a minimum of suffering and a maximum of benefit.

Offer everything you do to God (समर्पण)

If your occupation is honest, you can certainly conceive it as a work for God. Whether you are at a desk or doing housework, whatever the nature of your work, meditate on God. Offer to Him that you have done through the day, though it was apparently done for your employer. Have you typed twenty letters and taken them to him? Let him sign them, but afterwards close your eyes and offer all to the Lord. You will thus give a new turn to your thoughts. Yes, it is a different way of doing things. It may appear a little unusual at first but undertake it anyhow. Little by little a deeper meaning will be revealed, and you will find that this practice is not what you originally thought it to be; it will become tremendously effective.

In this way, whenever we do anything for others or for ourselves, we may think we are doing it for the Lord. Everything in life can then be converted into spiritual activity. There may be some who are able, consciously, and deliberately, to do things directly for God. How fortunate they are! That is why people perform elaborate worship. That is why they grow flowers and offer them on the altar, why they burn incense and light candles. Perhaps you do not like such practices? But how else would you spend the hours of the day? Don't you see that time and energy are wasted by serving the little self? Would it not be better to offer whatever you do to Him? Out of this feeling has come ritualism. Out of this feeling have been built temples, all over the world, where people bring offerings for worship.

However, it must be clarified that mere practise of ritualism is not being recommended. Each must worship according to his spiritual temperament. But in some manner, you will have to discover how to bring your own thoughts, emotions, and actions to the service of the Lord. The more you do it, the closer you will be to Him. Then, when you sit in meditation, everything else will be forgotten, and God alone will fill your heart.

Realise your true nature (आत्मज्ञान)

Perhaps we are accustomed to convincing ourselves of the reality of spiritual truths by means of reasoning. But until you have experienced these truths yourself, let me say that the greatest blessing would be for you to meet one who has realized them in person. You know, the proof of spiritual truths does not lie in reason, argument, or any kind of outward demonstration. Their proof lies in the sincere conviction carried by the words of a man who has realized what he expresses. Though others may disagree, I think that this is the one objective proof on which one can rely. If such an illumined person were to say to me, "My son, you are not really this body and mind; spirit is your true nature; the immortal and eternal being is the real you. Passing things do not belong to you. Try to penetrate the depths; try to realize your true self," I should be forced to accept and to act upon his words. As he spoke, something in his voice would sink deep into my heart; I should not be able to resist it. How I wish you could all find someone from whose lips such words would fall! You would not then be able to doubt or ignore them, and conviction of your true nature and glorious goal would grow within you. For a time, failure might cause you to despair, but eventually you would say, "All right, let me try again." And you would win. We have discussed what should be done preparatory to meditation. Your mind can be drawn ever closer to God by undertaking all the various measures that have been enumerated. In conclusion, a few points need to be stressed: Do whatever work is required of you but direct it to the Lord; then your mind will not be disturbed. Be unrelated. identify yourself with eternity; then meditation will be very easy. Do not let your mind wander, or worldly thoughts will enter and cloud it - this should never be permitted. Before you sit in meditation, think of the things suggested.

When nothing extraneous enters your mind, it will grow calm. Then, in the temple of your heart, you will begin to see the shining face of the Lord. Meditating upon it, you will find it more and more beautiful, and plunged in its infinite beauty, you will forget all else. You will at last be wholly absorbed in Him.

Ashtavakra Gita in chapter 15 verse 20, sums up the entire concept of meditational paradigm with thoughtless consciousness as follows.

tyajaiva dhyānaṃ sarvatra mā kiñciddhṛdi dhāraya |
ātmā tvaṃ mukta evāsi kiṃ vimṛśya kariṣyasi || 20 ||

"Give up all thoughts all around and keep nothing in your heart. You are pure consciousness, ever free and any form of contemplation will not serve any purpose"

CHAPTER FIVE

GYAN YOGA

Yoga in everyone's life.

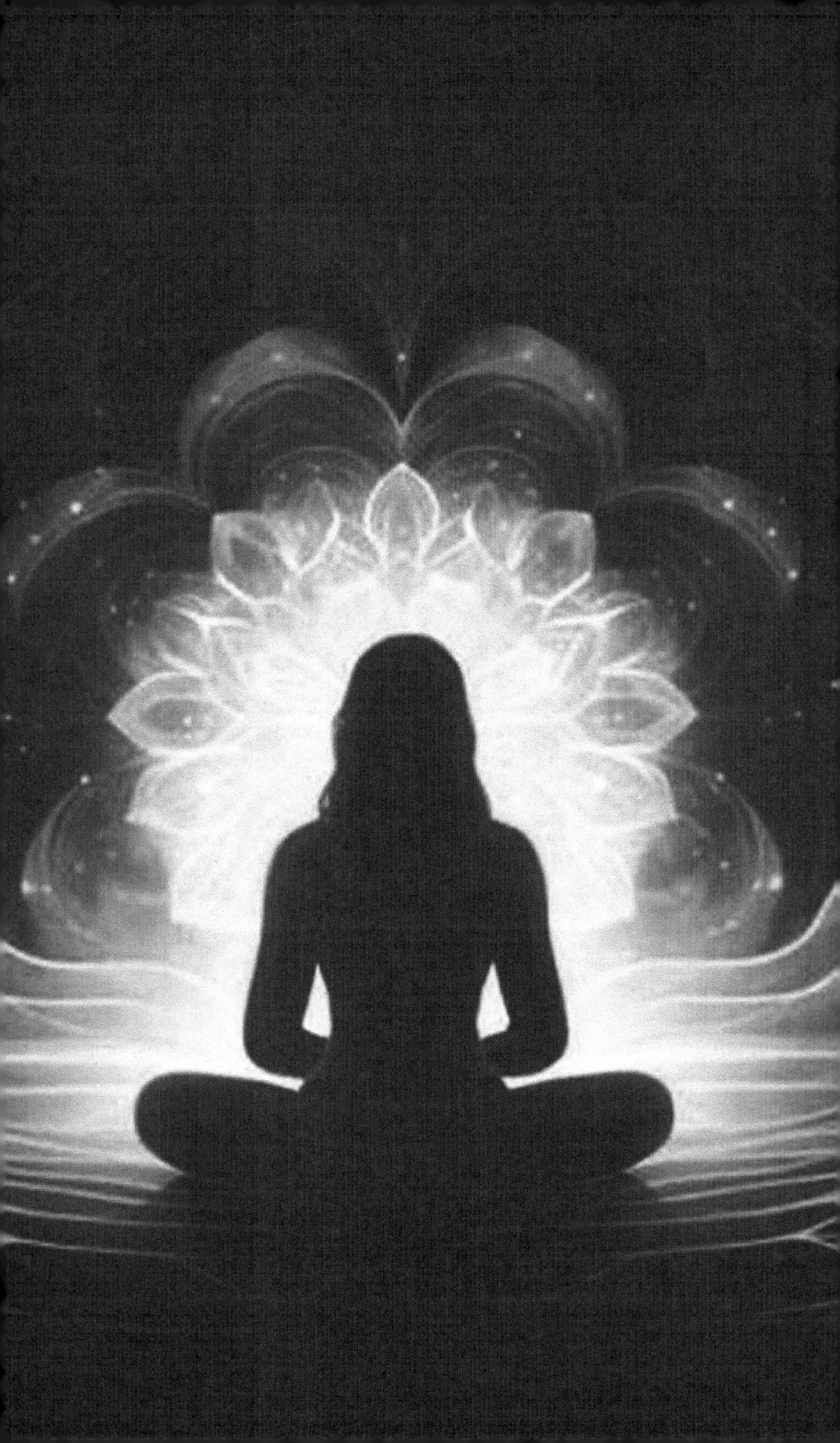

GYAAN YOGA

The highest a yogi can aspire for and indeed seek, is Gyan Yoga, the topmost rung of the ladder in his journey for liberation and God realization. He is just few steps away from achieving his goal. It is a long journey for all sentient beings because of deep seated error in understanding our true self. Cause of all errors is ignorance, and its removal is possible by knowledge. This is where the practice of Gyan Yoga becomes important. Truth is right there, but we are unable to see it clearly. It is like looking into the mirror which has been covered with dust and that prevents us from seeing our true face. We are right there but are unable to see our true self. Once the dust clears off, we get to see what we really are. Gyan Yoga helps to clear that dust, remove all impurities of head and heart, and reveals our true nature. One of the oft-repeated descriptions of an error in spiritual circles is confusing rope with a snake. A rope appears as a snake because of ignorance and once knowledge dawns the snake disappears, and rope can be seen in its true form.

Interestingly, what we really are is right there in front of us, but we fail to see it. There is a fascinating story of Mullah Nasrullah who was engaged in cross-border trade business. He would carry goods from one country to another and used donkeys to carry the stuff. At the border the security guards would stop him for checking whether he was doing anything illegal. They would check all the documents, and everything was always found in order. Nothing seemed amiss. He continued this practice for several years and in old age stopped doing it and retired. The chief of security also retired and met Mullah one day and asked him, "I always suspected that there was something not right in your dealings, but I could not pinpoint any irregularities. Now that I have retired, and you have stopped doing business, will you please tell me what is that you were taking inside illegally, if you were". Mullah was very candid and said of course, those were Donkeys that were being smuggled.

It is right there in front of our eyes, but we fail to see it. True Knowledge coupled with right discernment is the answer.

Nothing in this world is purer or purifying than knowledge. Krishna declares this with unequivocal firmness.

न हि ज्ञानेन सदृशं पवित्रमिह विद्यते |
तत्स्वयं योगसंसिद्धः कालेनात्मनि विन्दति || 38 ||

na hi jñānena sadṛiśhaṁ pavitramiha vidyate
tatsvayaṁ yogasansiddhaḥ kālenātmani vindati

na—not; hi—certainly; jñānena—with divine knowledge; sadriśham—like; pavitram—pure; iha—in this world; vidyate—exists; tat—that; svayam—oneself; yoga—practice of yog; sansiddhaḥ—he who has attained perfection; kālena—in course of time; ātmani—wihtin the heart; vindati—finds

In this world, there is nothing as purifying as divine knowledge. One who has attained purity of mind through prolonged practice of Yog, receives such knowledge within the heart, in due course of time.

Commentary

Knowledge has the power to purify, elevate, liberate, and unite a person with God. It is thus supremely sublime and pure. But a distinction needs to be made between two kinds of knowledge—theoretical information and practical realization.

There is one kind of knowledge that is acquired by reading the scriptures and hearing from the Guru. This theoretical information is insufficient by itself. It is just as if someone has memorized a cookbook but has never entered the kitchen. Such theoretical knowledge of cooking does not help in preparing a dish or satiating one's hunger. Similarly, one may acquire theoretical knowledge on the topics of the soul, God, Maya, *karm*, *jñāna*, and *bhakti* from the Guru, but that by itself does not make a person God-realized. When one practices *sādhanā* in accordance with the theory, it results in purification of the mind. Then, from within one gets realization of the nature of the self and its relationship with God. The Sage Patañjali states:

śhrutānumāna-prajñābhyām anya-viṣhayā viśheṣhārthatvāt
(Yog Darśhan 1.49) [v36]

"The knowledge attained by realization from within through the practice of Yog is far superior to theoretical knowledge of the scriptures." Such realized knowledge is being extolled by Shree Krishna as the purest sublime thing.

चतुर्विधा भजन्ते मां जनाः सुकृतिनोऽर्जुन ।
आर्तो जिज्ञासुरर्थार्थी ज्ञानी च भरतर्षभ ॥ 16 ॥ CH 7

chatur-vidhā bhajante māṁ janāḥ sukṛitino 'rjuna
ārto jijñāsur arthārthī jñānī cha bharatarṣhabha

chatuḥ-vidhāḥ—four kinds; bhajante—worship; mām—me; janāḥ—people; su-kritinaḥ—those who are pious; arjuna—Arjun; ārtaḥ—the distressed; jijñāsuḥ—the seekers of knowledge; artha-arthī—the seekers of material gain; jñānī—those who are situated in knowledge; cha—and; bharata-riṣhabha—The best amongst the Bharatas, Arjun

O best amongst the Bharatas, four kinds of pious people engage in My devotion—the distressed, the seekers of knowledge, the seekers of worldly possessions, and those who are situated in knowledge.

Commentary

In verse 15 of the chapter 7, Krishna described the four categories of people who do not surrender to Him. In verse 16, He describes; the other four kinds who take refuge in Him.

1. **The distressed.** Those who find that their pot of worldly miseries is overflowing, and they are unable to cope with them conclude that it is futile running after the world. Thus, decide to take shelter in God. Similarly, those who find that the worldly supports fail to protect them; turn to God for protection. An apt example in the Mahabharata was Draupadi's surrender to Krishna when Duryodhan and Dushasan tried to dishonour her in the courtroom of Hastinapur. Initially, she hoped her husbands would protect her, but they did not. She pleaded to the elders in the courtroom, Bheeshma, Vidur, Dhritarashtra, Dronacharya, Kripacharya, etc. However, everyone remained speechless and unmoved. When Dushasan tried to disrobe her, she clenched her sari with her teeth and tried to protect her honour with her own strength. But her teeth could not hold on to the sari for long; they gave in to Dushasan's strength. She was helpless and finally called out to Krishna for help. It was at this point that she surrendered completely to God and was not relying on anyone or her own strength for protection. Krishna responded immediately and intervened. Now, how much ever Dushasan pulled, Draupadi's sari kept extending, and very soon, there was a huge pile of cloth in the middle of the courtroom. Dushasan failed miserably in his attempt to disrobe Draupadi; exhausted, he gave up. Such was the power of God's protection, but it came only when Draupadi surrendered completely.

2. **The knowledge seekers.** There are some people who have heard about the opulence of God and His spiritual realm. Thus, they are curious to know all about God and try to seek Him through knowledge. (जिज्ञासु)

3. **The seekers of worldly possessions.** Some people are clear about what they want and take the shelter of God because they are convinced; that only God can provide what they are seeking. King Dhruv is an apt example. When Dhruv was a small boy, he felt neglected by his father, King Uttanapada. Disheartened, he went into the forest and did penance to please God. He wanted to become more powerful than his father. But as his devotion grew, he realized that God possessed the priceless jewel of divine love, and what he was seeking was like broken pieces of glass. Therefore, when pleased with his devotion, God gave him *darshan,* he requested the Lord to bestow upon him, self-less pure love.

4. **Those situated in knowledge.** Lastly, those souls who have understood the truth that they are just a small part of God. Such people engage in devotion with the intent that it is their eternal duty to love and serve Him. Krishna calls them the fourth kind of devotees.

तेषां ज्ञानी नित्ययुक्त एकभक्तिर्विशिष्यते |
प्रियो हि ज्ञानिनोऽत्यर्थमहं स च मम प्रियः || 17 || CH 7

teṣhāṁ jñānī nitya-yukta eka-bhaktir viśhiṣhyate
priyo hi jñānino 'tyartham ahaṁ sa cha mama priyaḥ

teṣhām—amongst these; jñānī—those who are situated in knowledge; nitya-yuktaḥ—ever steadfast; eka—exclusively; bhaktiḥ—devotion; viśhiṣhyate—highest; priyaḥ—very dear; hi—certainly; jñāninaḥ—to the person in knowledge; atyartham—highly; aham—I; saḥ—he; cha—and; mama—to me; priyaḥ—very dear

Amongst these, I consider them to be the highest, who worship Me with knowledge, and are steadfastly and exclusively devoted to Me. I am very dear to them, and they are very dear to Me.

Commentary

Krishan says in this verse that those who are seeking God in distress, for worldly gains or out of curiosity, etc. are yet to possess selfless devotion. Gradually in the process of devotion, their hearts become pure, and they realize their eternal relationship with God. Then they develop selfless, exclusive, and incessant devotion toward Him. Now that they have the knowledge that the happiness of the world is temporary and God is the source of eternal bliss, they neither crave for favourable circumstances nor lament over reversals in the world. They become situated in selfless devotion with complete self-surrender. And for their Divine Beloved, they are willing to offer themselves as an offering in the fire of divine love. Krishna declares that such devotees are dearest Him.

उदाराः सर्व एवैते ज्ञानी त्वात्मैव मे मतम् |
आस्थितः स हि युक्तात्मा मामेवानुत्तमां गतिम् || 18 ||CH 7

udārāḥ sarva evaite jñānī tvātmaiva me matam
āsthitaḥ sa hi yuktātmā mām evānuttamāṁ gatim

udārāḥ—noble; sarve—all; eva—indeed; ete—these; jñānī—those in knowledge; tu—but; ātmā eva—my very self; me—my; matam—opinion; āsthitaḥ—situated; saḥ—he; hi—certainly; yukta-ātmā—those who are united; mām—in me; eva—certainly; anuttamām—the supreme; gatim—goal

All those who are devoted to Me are indeed noble. But those in knowledge, who are of steadfast mind, whose intellect is merged in Me, and who have made Me alone as their supreme goal, I consider as my very self.

Commentary

In the previous verse, Krishna stated that the devotees situated in knowledge or *jñānī bhakt* are the highest. However, He clarifies in this verse that whatever may be the reason for their devotion, all His devotees are privileged; even the other three kinds are blessed souls. But the devotees seated in knowledge worship God selflessly, without expecting any material gains in return. Hence, the unconditional love of such selfless devotees even binds God.

Worldly love; is driven by the desire for self-gratification. There is a give and take attitude, and there is an expectation of receiving something in return from the beloved. However, *Parā bhakti* or divine love is totally different. It is filled with the desire for the happiness of the Divine Beloved and sacrifice in His service. Divine love fosters an attitude of selflessness without expecting anything in return.

Chaitanya Mahaprabhu said:

kāmera tātparya nija-sambhoga kevala
kṛiṣhṇa-sukha-tātparya-mātra prema ta' prabala

ataeva kāma-preme bahuta antara
kāma andha-tamaḥ, prema nirmala bhāskara
(Chaitanya Charitāmṛit, Ādi Leela, 4.166 & 171) [v16]

"Lust (worldly love) exists for self-happiness; divine love is harboured for Krishna's happiness. There is a tremendous difference between them—lust is like darkness and ignorance, while divine love is pure and illuminating."

brahma lok paryanta sukh, aru muktihuñ sukh tyāg,
tabai dharahu paga prema patha, nahiṅ lagi jaiheñ dāg.
(Bhakti Śhatak verse 45) [v17]

"Give up the desires for worldly pleasures and that of liberation if you wish to walk the path of devotion. Else the pure waters of divine love will get tainted with selfishness."

Sage Narad defined pure devotion in this manner:

tat sukha sukhitvam (Nārad Bhakti Darśhan, Sūtra 24)[v18]

"True love is for the happiness of the Beloved." The materially motivated devotees cannot engage in such devotion, but the devotee who is in knowledge rises to this level of selflessness. When someone learns to love God in this manner, He becomes a slave of that Devotee. The highest quality of God is *bhakta vatsaltā* (his love for his devotees).

The Puraṇas state:

gītvā cha mama nāmāni vicharenmama sannidhau
iti bravīmi te satyaṁ krītohaṁ tasya chārjuna
(Ādi Purāṇ 1.2.231) [v19]

Krishna says: "I become the slave of those devotees of mine, who chant my names and keep me close to them in their thoughts; this is a fact, O Arjun."

In this verse Krishna goes to the extent of saying that bound by the devotion and love of His selfless devotees, He looks upon them as Himself.

श्रद्धावान् लभते ज्ञानं तत्परः संयतेन्द्रियः |
ज्ञानं लब्ध्वा परां शान्तिमचिरेणाधिगच्छति || 39 || CH 4

śhraddhāvānllabhate jñānaṁ tat-paraḥ sanyatendriyaḥ
jñānaṁ labdhvā parāṁ śhāntim achireṇādhigachchhati

śhraddhāvān—a faithful person; labhate—achieves; jñānam—divine knowledge; tat-paraḥ—devoted (to that); sanyata—controlled; indriyaḥ—senses; jñānam—transcendental knowledge; labdhvā—having achieved; parām—supreme; śhāntim—peace; achireṇa—without delay; adhigachchhati—attains

Those whose faith is deep and who have practiced controlling their mind and senses attain divine knowledge. Through such transcendental knowledge, they quickly attain everlasting supreme peace.

Commentary

Krishna now introduces the concept of faith in the context of knowledge. Not all spiritual truths are immediately perceptible; some of them can only be experienced after having attained sufficient elevation on the path. If we only accept what we can presently verify or comprehend, we will be bereft of the higher spiritual secrets. Faith helps us accept what we cannot understand at present. Jagadguru Shankaracharya has defined faith as follows:

guru vedānta vākyeṣhu dṛiḍho viśhvāsaḥ śhraddhā [v37]

"Faith means firm confidence in the words of the Guru and the scriptures." When such faith is placed upon a wrong personality, it can lead to disastrous consequences. But when it is placed on the true Guru, it opens the pathway for eternal welfare.

However, blind faith is not a desirable thing. Before placing it on any Guru, we must use our intellect to confirm that the Guru has realized the Absolute Truth, and he is teaching it in accordance with the eternal Vedic scriptures. Once this is confirmed, then we should strive to deepen our faith in such a Guru and surrender to God under his guidance. The Shvetashvatar Upaniṣhad states:

yasya deve parā bhaktir yathā deve tathā gurau
tasyaite kathitā hyarthāḥ prakāśhante mahātmanaḥ
(6.23) [v38]

"The imports of all the Vedic knowledge are revealed within the hearts of those who engage with unflinching faith in devotion toward Guru and God."

सत्त्वानुरूपा सर्वस्य श्रद्धा भवति भारत |
श्रद्धामयोऽयं पुरुषो यो यच्छ्रद्धः स एव सः || 3 || CH 17

sattvānurūpā sarvasya śhraddhā bhavati bhārata
śhraddhā-mayo 'yaṁ puruṣho yo yach-chhraddhaḥ sa eva saḥ

sattva-anurūpā—conforming to the nature of one's mind; sarvasya—all; śhraddhā—faith; bhavati—is; bhārata—Arjun, the scion of Bharat; śhraddhāmayah—possessing faith; ayam—that; puruṣhah—human being; yaḥ—who; yat-śhraddhaḥ—whatever the nature of their faith; saḥ—their; eva—verily; saḥ—they

The faith of all humans conforms to the nature of their mind. All people possess faith, and whatever the nature of their faith, that is verily what they are.

Commentary

In the previous verse, it was explained that we all repose our faith somewhere or the other. Where we decide to place our faith and what we choose to believe in practically shapes the direction of our life. Those who develop the conviction that money is of paramount importance in the world spend their entire life accumulating it. Those who believe that fame counts more than anything else dedicate their time and energy in chasing political posts and social designations. Those who believe in noble values, sacrifice everything to uphold them. Mahatma Gandhi had faith in the incomparable importance of *satya* (truth) and *ahinsā* (non-violence), and by the strength of his convictions he launched a non-violent movement that succeeded in evicting from India the most powerful empire in the world. Those who develop deep faith in the overriding importance of God-realization renounce their material life in search of him. Thus, Shree Krishna states that the quality of our faith decides the direction of our life. In turn, the quality of our faith is decided by the nature of our mind.

Knowledge is one of the most widely used word and has a strong connect with the truth which really is the fundamental need of all civilizations down the ages. Everyone must know the world one is born in. No one comes into the world of his or her own volition. Having come to the world, or more correctly, having been born, one wants to live and live happily and productively. Interestingly, one does not want to leave the world on his own volition. Be that as it may, everyone wants to live and evolve and for that one needs knowledge, one needs to learn the art of survival first, and then the art of living.

Knowledge is as vast as it is the fundamental to the entire existence and its structure is ensconced in the science of epistemology. It is the philosophical study of the nature, origin, and limits of human knowledge. The term epistemology is derived from the Greek episteme (knowledge) and logos (reason) and the field is often referred to as the theory of knowledge. It explores various parameters and concepts, and it would be worthwhile to describe some of the significant ones.

1. Epistemology examines what knowledge is and how it can be acquired, justified, or defined.

2. It explores the nature of belief and its role in forming knowledge. How are beliefs formed, justified, and changed.

3. Epistemology seeks to understand the nature of the truth and how it relates to knowledge. What does it mean for a belief or a proposition to be true?

4. This parameter focuses on the methods or criteria used to justify beliefs or claims to knowledge. How can we provide reasonable grounds or evidence for what we claim to know?

5. Epistemology often grapples with scepticism, which challenges the possibility or limits of knowledge. It challenges whether certain knowledge is attainable or if we can acquire it with the acceptable means.

6. It dwells upon the reasoning processes involved in acquiring and evaluating knowledge. How can we use reason and logic to reach justified beliefs?

7. Epistemology investigates the roles of empirical experience and rational thought in acquiring knowledge. Is knowledge primarily derived from direct sensory experience or requires corroboration by other means including observation? To get a better understanding of Gyan Yoga, it would also be necessary to look closely at the tenets of ontology which is

a branch of metaphysics dealing with study of beings, existence, and reality. Ontology is specifically the study of existence and its nature. Theories within ontology are theories that explain the nature of existence by describing its substance or causes. At its core, ontology is the study of 'what is'. To make this little more concrete, one could also say ontology is the study of what exists or what is real. “Does God exist? “Are my feelings real?' What is nothing” and “does it exist”; are all examples of ontological questions.

The science of epistemology and ontology has a direct bearing on the concept and practice of Gyan Yoga. The basic question that all of us grapple with, is to know about the universe, about ourselves, why are we here? What is the purpose of our life? Do we die with the death of the body? Is there something called Soul which is eternal and imperishable? Is there a phenomenon called Rebirth?

Modern science, scientific investigations do not have any clear answer to these and related questions. However, some of the recent path breaking discoveries in Physics, Chemistry, and biology, coupled with newer knowledge in the field of neurosciences have aroused the interests of several scientists and philosophers worldwide, and study of Consciousness has attracted the attention of many.

Interestingly, ancient Indian thought, Vedas, body of Upanishads, especially Advaita Vedanta have answers on these questions and the West has started looking eastwards for enlightenment.

Gyan Yoga essentially, is a study of the Self and our relationship with Nature, its creator, and our goal of life. Everyone who is born must die, some sooner, some later and what should, or how should we do what we do, during that interregnum. We have no control on our birth, we do not control our time and cause of death. However, in between we must manage. All living beings are organic entities and inherent in their intrinsic structure is birth, growth, development, maturity, decay, and death. This process is immutable and there are no exceptions-not even one. One important question to which everyone seeks an answer, relates to our absolute disappearance from the earth, or whether something in us survives and is renewed in another living form.

Bhagavad-Gita has clear answers to these questions. Arjuna experiences irremovable bouts of depression at the thought of killing his own dear and near ones, including his Gurus, Grandfather, friends, and relations in the battlefield of Mahabharata. He obdurately refuses to pick up his bow and arrows, and no amount of cajoling and persuasion by Krishna made him change his mind. Krishna faced a huge dilemma. He knew that the only person, who could be instrumental in fulfilling the objective of His appearance (Avatar) in the world in human form, was Arjuna, the great warrior. On his own statement, Krishna declares that whenever there is a decline of values in the social fabric, when evil forces prevail over goodness, He appears in this world to restore the reign of good over evil and give protection to the oppressed.

Krishna then explains the eternal nature of all living beings. Not of the body, which is perishable, and goes through several stages of birth, decay, and death, but of the soul/consciousness which is imperishable. At one place, He says that the soul cannot be slayed by the sword, is not burnt by fire. Even water cannot make it wet, nor the breeze can make it dry.

नैनं छिन्दन्ति शस्त्राणि नैनं दहति पावकः |
न चैनं क्लेदयन्त्यापो न शोषयति मारुतः || 23 ||

nainaṁ chhindanti śhastrāṇi nainaṁ dahati pāvakaḥ
na chainaṁ kledayantyāpo na śhoṣhayati mārutaḥ

na—not; enam—this soul; chhindanti—shred; śhastrāṇi—weapons; na—nor; enam—this soul; dahati—burns; pāvakaḥ—fire; na—not; cha—and; enam—this soul; kledayanti—moisten; āpaḥ—water; na—nor; śhoṣhayati—dry; mārutaḥ—wind

Translation

Weapons cannot shred the soul, nor can fire burn it. Water cannot wet it, nor can the wind dry it.

Commentary

Consciousness, which is the symptom of the soul, can be perceived by material instruments, but the soul itself cannot be contacted by any material object. This is so only because the soul is divine, and hence beyond the interactions of material objects. Shree Krishna expresses this vividly by saying that wind cannot wither the soul, nor can water moisten it or fire burn it.

Disabusing Arjuna's mind completely of his being responsible for killing anybody, He says that all those who are present in the battlefield will never go away. You, all those you see, and I, have had several births. I know about all of them-you don't.

श्रीभगवानुवाच |
बहूनि मे व्यतीतानि जन्मानि तव चार्जुन |
तान्यहं वेद सर्वाणि न त्वं वेत्थ परन्तप || 5 || CH 4

śhrī bhagavān uvācha
bahūni me vyatītāni janmāni tava chārjuna
tānyahaṁ veda sarvāṇi na tvaṁ vettha parantapa

śhrī-bhagavān uvācha—the Supreme Lord said; bahūni—many; me—of mine; vyatītāni—have passed; janmāni—births; tava—of yours; cha—and; arjuna—Arjun; tāni—them; aham—I; veda—know; sarvāṇi—all; na—not; tvam—you; vettha—know; parantapa—Arjun, the scorcher of foes

Translation

The Supreme Lord said: Both you and I have had many births, O Arjun. You have forgotten them, while I remember them all, O Parantapa.

Commentary

Krishna explains that merely because he is standing before Arjun in the human form, he should not be equated with human beings. The president of a country sometimes decides to visit the prison, but if we see the president standing in the jail, we do not erroneously conclude that he is also a convict. We know that he is in the jail merely for an inspection. Similarly, God sometimes descends in the material world, but he is never divested of his divine attributes and powers.

In his commentary upon this verse, Shankaracharya states: *yā vāsudeve anīśhvarāsarvajñāśhaṅkā mūrkhāṇāṁ tāṁ pariharan śhrī-bhagavān uvācha* (*Śhārīrak Bhāṣhya* on verse 4.5) [v2]

"This verse has been spoken by Krishna to explain to the ignorant who doubt that he is God." Non-believers argue that Krishna too was born like the rest of us, and he ate, drank, slept, like we all do, and so he could not have been God. Here, Krishna emphasizes the difference between the soul and God by stating that although he descends in the world innumerable times, he remains omniscient, unlike the soul whose knowledge is finite.

The individual soul and the Supreme Soul, God, have many similarities—both are *sat-chit-ānand* (eternal, sentient, and blissful). However, there are also many differences. God is all-pervading, while the soul only pervades the body it inhabits; God is all-powerful, while the soul does not even have the power to liberate itself from Maya without God's grace; God is the creator of the laws of nature, while the soul is subject to these laws; God is the upholder of the entire creation, while the soul is upheld by him; God is all-knowing, while the soul does not have complete knowledge even in one subject.

Krishna calls Arjun in this verse as "Parantapa," meaning "subduer of the enemies." He implies, "Arjun, you are a valiant warrior who has slayed so many powerful enemies. Now, do not accept defeat influenced by the doubt that has crept in your mind. Use the sword of knowledge to slay your foes and be situated in wisdom."

Further elaborating on the eternal nature of the soul, He tells Arjuna that all those you see in front of you, were always present and will always be there. You don't need to grieve over their physical disappearance.

न त्वेवाहं जातु नासं न त्वं नेमे जनाधिपाः |
न चैव न भविष्यामः सर्वे वयमतः परम् || 12 || CH 2

na tvevāhaṁ jātu nāsaṁ na tvaṁ neme janādhipāḥ
na chaiva na bhaviṣhyāmaḥ sarve vayamataḥ param

na—never; tu—however; eva—certainly; aham—I; jātu—at any time; na—nor; āsam—exist; na—nor; tvam—you; na—nor; ime—these; jana-adhipāḥ—kings; na—never; cha—also; eva—indeed; na bhaviṣhyāmaḥ—shall not exist; sarve vayam—all of us; ataḥ—from now; param—after

Never was there a time when I did not exist, nor you, nor all these kings; nor in the future shall any of us cease to be.

Commentary

On the gate of the temple of Apollo at Delphi are inscribed the words, *Gnothi Seuton*, or "Know Thyself [v8]." Even Socrates, the wise old man of Athens, was fond of encouraging people to inquire into the nature of the self. A local legend goes like this. Once, Socrates was walking on the street, absorbed in deep philosophic contemplation, when he accidentally bumped into someone. That man blurted in annoyance, "Can't you see where you walk? Who are you?" Socrates answered with amusement, "My dear fellow, I have been pondering over that question for the last forty years. If you ever come to know who I am, please let me know."

In the Vedic tradition, whenever divine knowledge is imparted, it usually begins with knowledge of the self. Krishna follows the same approach in the **Bhagavad Gita**, with a piece of information that would have swept Socrates off his feet. Shree Krishna begins by explaining that the entity that we call the "self" is really the soul, not the material body, and is eternal, just as God himself is eternal. The Śhwetāśhvatar Upaniṣhad states:

jñājñau dwāvajā vīśhanīśhāvajā hyekā bhoktṛi bhogyārtha yuktā
anantaśhchātmā viśhwarūpo hyakartā trayaṁ yadā vindate brahmametat
(1.9) [v9]

The above verse states that creation is a combination of three entities—God, soul, and Maya—and all the three entities are eternal. *If we believe the soul is eternal, then it follows logically that there is life after death of the material body. Krishna talks about this in the next verse.*

देहिनोऽस्मिन्यथा देहे कौमारं यौवनं जरा |
तथा देहान्तरप्राप्तिर्धीरस्तत्र न मुह्यति || 13 || CH 2

dehino 'smin yathā dehe kaumāraṁ yauvanaṁ jarā
tathā dehāntara-prāptir dhīras tatra na muhyati

dehinaḥ—of the embodied; asmin—in this; yathā—as; dehe—in the similarly; deha-antara—another body; prāptiḥ—achieves; dhīraḥ—the wise; tatra—thereupon; na muhyati—are not deluded

Just as the embodied soul continuously passes from childhood to youth to old age, similarly, at the time of death, the soul passes into another body. The wise are not deluded by this.

Commentary

With immaculate logic, Krishna establishes the principle of transmigration of the soul from lifetime to lifetime. He explains that in one lifetime itself, we change bodies from childhood to youth to maturity and then to old age. In fact, modern science informs us that cells within the body undergo regeneration—old cells die away, and new ones take their place. It is estimated that within seven years, practically all the cells of the body change. Further, the molecules within the cells change even more rapidly. With every breath we inhale, oxygen molecules are absorbed into our cells via the metabolic processes, and molecules that were heretofore locked within the cells are released as carbon dioxide. Scientists estimate that in one year's time, about ninety-eight percent of our bodily molecules change. And yet, despite the continual change of the body, we perceive that we are the same person. That is because we are not the material body, but the spiritual soul seated within.

In this verse, the word *deha* means "the body" and *dehi* means "possessor of the body," or the soul. Krishna draws Arjun's attention to the fact that, since the body is constantly changing, in one lifetime itself, the soul passes through many bodies. Similarly, at the time of death, it passes into another body. What we term as "death" in worldly parlance is merely the soul discarding its old dysfunctional body, and what we call "birth" is the soul taking on a new body elsewhere. This is the principle of reincarnation.

Most Oriental philosophies accept this concept of reincarnation. It is an integral part of Hinduism, Jainism, and Sikhism. In Buddhism, the Buddha made references to his past lives repeatedly. Many people do not know the extent to which reincarnation was a part of the belief system of the Occidental philosophies as well. In ancient classical Western religious and philosophic circles, famous thinkers such as Pythagoras, Plato, and Socrates accepted reincarnation to be true, and their views were also reflected in Orphism, Hermeticism, Neoplatonism, Manicheanism, and Gnosticism. Within the mainstream Abrahamic faiths, mystics of the three major religions also supported reincarnation. Examples include Jews who studied the Kabbalah, the Christian Cathars, and Muslim Shia sects such as the Alawi Shias and the Druze. For example, amongst Occidental religions, Josephus, the great ancient Jewish historian, used language in his writings that seem to ascribe belief in some form of reincarnation among the Pharisees and Essenes of his day. Certainly, the Jewish Kabbalah prescribes to the idea of reincarnation as gilgul neshamot, or the "rolling of the soul." The great Sufi mystic, Maulana Jalaluddin Rumi declared:

I died out of the stone, and I became a plant;
I died out of the plant and became an animal;
I died out of the animal and became a man.
Why then should I fear to die?
When did I grow less by dying?
I shall die out of man and shall become an angel!" [v10]

Many of the early Christians believed in the concept of reincarnation. Christian history informs us that, in the 553 AD, the Council of Nicaea, a conclave, was held to discuss the principle of reincarnation, and it was thereafter declared a heresy, apparently to increase the authority of the Church over the lives of the people. Until then, it was commonly accepted. Jesus indirectly proclaimed this doctrine when he told his disciples that John the Baptist was Elijah the Prophet reincarnated (Matthew 11:13-14, Matthew 17:10-13). This is also mentioned in the Old Testament (Malachi 4:5). Origen, the most learned of the Christian Fathers, declared: "Every man receives a body for himself according to his deserts in former lives [v11]." Solomon's Book of Wisdom says: "To be born in sound body with sound limbs is a reward of the virtues of the past lives." (Wisdom of Solomon 8:19-20) [v12]

Belief in reincarnation is also found in many tribal societies around the world, in places such as Siberia, West Africa, North America, and Australia. Moving to more recent centuries and civilizations, reincarnation has been affirmed by Rosicrucian's, Spiritism, Theosophists, and New Age followers. Even more recently, it has even been studied in serious scientific circles at major universities, exemplified by the works of Dr. Ian Stevenson and Dr. Jim Tucker, both at the University of Virginia.

Without accepting the concept of rebirth, it is difficult to make sense out of the suffering, chaos, and incompleteness of the world, and hence, many famous western thinkers believed in this principle. Virgil and Ovid regarded this doctrine as self-evident. The German philosophers Goethe, Fichte, Schelling, and Lessing accepted it. Amongst the more recent philosophers, Hume, Spencer, and Max Mueller, all recognized it as an incontrovertible doctrine. Among Western poets, Browing, Rosetti, Tennyson, and Wordsworth, to mention just a few, all believed in it.

Krishna has previously declared that the wise do not lament. But the fact remains that we do experience happiness and distress. What is the reason for it? He now explains this concept.

While assertions made by Krishna in Bhagwat-Gita should be a conclusive proof of the eternal nature of all beings, we must further examine it with some more evidence which would be essentially experiential and inferential. It must be observed that there cannot be any direct proof of this fact because of the limits of our own sensory/intellectual perceptions, through which we ordinarily acquire knowledge. Additionally, Vedanta and all scriptures including Bhagwat-Gita describe God as Nirguna/Nirankar, an extremely subtle entity without any shape and attribute. God is also known to be omnipresent-present everywhere by all faiths and ideologies. Axiomatically speaking, something which is everywhere cannot be seen anywhere. Presence of air is experienced by everyone but is not seen anywhere. This is a direct experiential statement and cannot be disputed by any rational being. Chapter 13 of Gita makes some categorical statements in this regard.

सर्वेन्द्रियगुणाभासं सर्वेन्द्रियविवर्जितम् |
असक्तं सर्वभृच्चैव निर्गुणं गुणभोक्तृ च || 15 || CH 13

sarvendriya-guṇābhāsaṁ sarvendriya-vivarjitam
asaktaṁ sarva-bhṛich chaiva nirguṇaṁ guṇa-bhoktṛi cha

sarva—all; indriya—senses; guna—sense-objects; ābhāsam—the perciever; sarva—all; indriya—senses; vivarjitam—devoid of; asaktam—unattached; sarva-bhṛit—the sustainer of all; cha—yet; eva—indeed; nirguṇam—beyond the three modes of material nature; guṇa-bhoktṛi—the enjoyer of the three modes of material nature; cha—although

Though He perceives all sense-objects, yet He is devoid of the senses. He is unattached to everything, and yet He is the sustainer of all. Although He is without attributes, yet He is the enjoyer of the three modes of material nature.

Commentary

Having stated that God's senses are everywhere, Krishna now states the exact opposite, that He does not possess any senses. If we try to understand this through mundane logic, we will find this contradictory. We will inquire, "How can God have both infinite senses and also be without senses?" However, mundane logic does not apply to Him who is beyond the reach of the intellect. God possesses infinite contradictory attributes at the same time.

The Brahma Vaivarta Purāṇ states:
viruddha dharmo rūposā vaiśhvaryāt puruṣhottamāh

"The Supreme Lord is the reservoir of innumerable contradictory attributes." In this verse, Krishna mentions a few of the infinite contradictory attributes that exist in the personality of God.

He is devoid of mundane senses like ours, and hence it is correct to say that He does not have senses. *Sarvendriya vivarjitam* means "He is without material senses." However, He possesses divine senses that are everywhere, consequently, it is also correct to say that the senses of God are in all places. *Sarvendriya guṇābhāsaṁ* means "He manifests the functions of the senses and grasps the sense objects." Including both these attributes, the Śhwetāśhvatar Upaniṣhad states:

apāṇipādo javano grahītā, paśhyatyachakṣhuḥ sa śhṛiṇotyakarṇaḥ (3.19)

"God does not possess material hands, feet, eyes, and ears. Yet He grasps, walks, sees, and hears."

Further, Krishna states that He is the sustainer of creation, and yet detached from it. In His form as Lord Vishnu, God maintains the entire creation. He sits in the hearts of all living beings, notes their karmas, and gives the results. Under Lord Vishnu's dominion, Brahma manipulates the laws of material science to ensure that the universe functions stably. Also, under Lord Vishnu's dominion, the celestial gods arrange to provide the air, earth, water, rain, etc. that are necessary for our survival. Hence, God is the Sustainer of all. Yet, He is complete in Himself and is, thus, detached from everyone. The Vedas mention Him as *ātmārām*, meaning "one who rejoices in the self and has no need of anything external."

The material energy is subservient to God, and it works for His pleasure by serving Him. He is thus the enjoyer of the three *guṇas* (modes of material nature). At the same time, He is also *nirguṇa* (beyond the three *guṇas*), because these *guṇas* are material, while God is divine.

यदा भूतपृथग्भावमेकस्थमनुपश्यति |
तत एव च विस्तारं ब्रह्म सम्पद्यते तदा || 31 || CH 13

yadā bhūta-pṛithag-bhāvam eka-stham anupaśhyati
tata eva cha vistāraṁ brahma sampadyate tadā

yadā—when; bhūta—living entities; prithak-bhāvam—diverse variety; eka-stham—situated in the same place; anupaśhyati—see; tataḥ—thereafter; eva—indeed; cha—and; vistāram—born from; brahma—Brahman; sampadyate—(they) attain; tadā—then

When they see the diverse variety of living beings situated in the same material nature and understand all of them to be born from it, they attain the realization of the Brahman.

Commentary

The ocean modifies itself in many forms such as the wave, froth, tide, ripples, etc. One who is shown all these individually for the first time may conclude that they are all different. But one who has knowledge of the ocean sees the inherent unity in all the variety. Similarly, there are numerous forms of life in existence, from the tiniest amoeba to the most powerful celestial gods. All of them are rooted in the same reality—the soul, which is a part of God, seated in a body, which is made from the material energy. The distinctions between the forms are not due to the soul, but due to the different bodies manifested by the material energy. Upon birth, the bodies of all living beings are created from the material energy, and at death, their bodies again merge into it. When we see the variety of living beings all rooted in the same material nature, we realize the unity behind the diversity. And since material nature is the energy of God, such an understanding makes us see the same spiritual substratum pervading all existence. This leads to the Brahman realization.

अनादित्वान्निर्गुणत्वात्परमात्मायमव्ययः |
शरीरस्थोऽपि कौन्तेय न करोति न लिप्यते || 32 || CH 13

anāditvān nirguṇatvāt paramātmāyam avyayaḥ
śharīra-stho 'pi kaunteya na karoti na lipyate

anāditvāt—being without beginning; nirguṇatvāt—being devoid of any material qualities; parama—the Supreme; ātmā—soul; ayam—this; avyayaḥ—imperishable; śharīra-sthaḥ—dwelling in the body; api—although; kaunteya—Arjun, the the son of Kunti; na—neither; karoti—acts; na—nor; lipyate—is tainted

The Supreme Soul is imperishable, without beginning, and devoid of any material qualities, O son of Kunti. Although situated within the body, it neither acts, nor is It tainted by material energy.

Commentary

God, situated within the heart of the living being as the Supreme Soul, never identifies with the body, nor is affected by its states of existence. His presence in the material body does not make Him material in any way, nor is He subject to the law of karma and the cycle of birth and death, though these are experienced by the soul.

यथा सर्वगतं सौक्ष्म्यादाकाशं नोपलिप्यते |
सर्वत्रावस्थितो देहे तथात्मा नोपलिप्यते || 33 || CH 13

yathā sarva-gataṁ saukṣhmyād ākāśhaṁ nopalipyate
sarvatrāvasthito dehe tathātmā nopalipyate

yathā—as; sarva-gatam—all-pervading; saukṣhmyāt—due to subtlety; ākāśham—the space; na—not; upalipyate—is contaminated; sarvatra—everywhere; avasthitaḥ—situated; dehe—the body; tathā—similarly; ātmā—the soul; na—not; upalipyate—is contaminated

Space holds everything within it, but being subtle, does not get contaminated by what it holds. Similarly, though its consciousness pervades the body, the soul is not affected by the attributes of the body.

Commentary

The soul experiences sleep, waking, tiredness, refreshment, etc., due to the ego that makes it identify with the body. One may ask why changes in the body in which it resides do not taint the soul. Krishna explains it with the example of space. It holds everything, yet remains unaffected, because it is subtler than the gross objects it holds. Similarly, the soul is a subtler energy. It retains Its divinity even while it identifies with the material body.

यथा प्रकाशयत्येक: कृत्स्नं लोकमिमं रवि: |
क्षेत्रं क्षेत्री तथा कृत्स्नं प्रकाशयति भारत || 34 || CH 13

yathā prakāśhayaty ekaḥ kṛitsnaṁ lokam imaṁ raviḥ
kṣhetraṁ kṣhetrī tathā kṛitsnaṁ prakāśhayati bhārata

yathā—as; prakāśhayati—illumines; ekaḥ—one; kṛitsnam—entire; lokam—solar system; imam—this; raviḥ—sun; kṣhetram—the body; kṣhetrī—the soul; tathā—so; kṛitsnam—entire; prakāśhayati—illumine; bhārata—Arjun, the son of Bharat

Just as one sun illumines the entire solar system, so does the individual soul illumine the entire body (with consciousness).

Commentary

Although the soul energizes the entire body in which it is present with consciousness, yet by itself, it is exceedingly small. *eṣho 'ṇurātmā* (Muṇḍakopaniṣhad 3.1.9) "The soul is very tiny in size." The Śhwetāśhvatar Upaniṣhad states:

bālāgraśhatabhāgasya śhatadhā kalpitasya cha
bhāgo jīvaḥ sa vijñeyaḥ sa chānantyāya kalpate (5.9)

"If we divide the tip of a hair into a hundred parts, and then divide each part into further hundred parts, we will get the size of the soul. These souls are innumerable in number." This is a manner of expressing the minuteness of the soul.

How can such an infinitesimal soul energize the body, which is huge in comparison? Krishna explains this with the analogy of the sun. Although situated in one place, the sun illumines the entire solar system with its light. Likewise, the Vedānt Darśhan states:

guṇādvā lokavat (2.3.25)

"The soul, although seated in the heart spreads its consciousness throughout the field of the body."

We will closely enumerate essential features of two branches of ancient philosophical thought that evolved since the beginning of civilization. Four Vedas, indisputably the oldest scriptures known to mankind are the most profound repository of knowledge. Literal translation of the word Veda is Knowledge, to know, sacred writings. In fact, wise ones interpret the meaning of the word further to mean- "All that is there is to know". In other words, the entire knowledge is encapsulated in Vedas and from them into Upanishads. (वेद नाम उपनिषद प्रमाण)

The philosophy of Samkhya Yoga was enunciated by Sage Kapila. Swami Vivekananda calls him the first philosopher of human race. It recognises the existence of Prakriti and Purusha as parallel entities, ever since the beginning of the universe, having been created by God and verily in existence ever since God existed. Prakriti is the material nature as we see it-the world, rivers, oceans, mountains, air, water, fire, sky, and earth. All that is gross and visible falls under the purview of Prakriti. It is also the cause of three Gunas-Satvik, Rajasic and Tamasic. These three Gunas, drive all actions of all creations and generate corresponding energy in the universe that eventually impact the evolutionary process. No one in this world is free from these Gunas that are present in every creature in different measure. Prevalence of one of these three builds one's reputation.

न तदस्ति पृथिव्यां वा दिवि देवेषु वा पुनः |
सत्त्वं प्रकृतिजैर्मुक्तं यदेभिः स्यात्त्रिभिर्गुणैः || 40 ||

na tad asti pṛithivyāṁ vā divi deveṣhu vā punaḥ
sattvaṁ prakṛiti-jair muktaṁ yad ebhiḥ syāt tribhir guṇaiḥ

na—no; tat—that; asti—exists; pṛithivyām—on earth; vā—or; divi—the higher celestial abodes; deveṣhu—amongst the celestial gods; vā—or; punaḥ—again; sattvam—existence; prakṛiti-jaiḥ—born of material nature; muktam—liberated; yat—that; ebhiḥ—from the influence of these; syāt—is; tribhiḥ—three; guṇaiḥ—modes of material nature

No living being on earth, or the higher celestial abodes of this material realm is free from the influence of these three modes of nature.

Commentary

The Śhwetāśhvatar Upaniṣhad states that the material energy, Maya, is tri-colored:

ajāmekāṁ lohita-śhukla-kṛiṣhṇāṁ bahvīḥ prajāḥ sṛijamānāṁ sa-rūpāḥ
ajo hy eko juṣhamāṇo 'nuśhete jahāty enāṁ bhukta-bhogām ajo
'nyaḥ...(4.5) [v22]

"Material nature has three colours—white, red, and black, i.e., it has three modes—goodness, passion, and ignorance. It is the mother-like womb of the innumerable living beings within the universe. It is brought into existence and supported by the one unborn Lord, who is full of knowledge. God, however, does not consort with his material energy. He independently enjoys the pleasure of his transcendental pastimes. But the living entity enjoys her and thus becomes bound."

Maya's domain extends from the nether regions to the celestial abode of Brahma. Since the three modes of nature—*sattva, rajas,* and *tamas*—are inherent attributes of Maya, they exist in all the material abodes of existence. Hence all living beings in these abodes, be they humans or the celestial gods, are under the sway of these three modes. The difference is only in the relative proportions of the three *guṇas*. The residents of the nether regions have a predominance of *tamas*; the residents of the earth planet have a predominance of *rajas*; and the residents of the celestial abodes have a predominance of *sattva*. Now, using these three variables, Krishna explains why human beings possess differing natures.

While Prakriti itself is eternal, the object created by its Maya are transient in nature and hence perishable.

Ashtavakra Gita the most radical scripture of Advaita Vedanta in chapter 1 verse 18, in response to a question by King Janak says.

sākāramanṛtaṃ viddhi nirākāraṃ tu niścalam |
etattattvopadeśena na punarbhavasaṃbhavaḥ || 18 ||

"You must know that whatever takes form is false. Only the formless is permanent. On realising this, you will escape the pangs of rebirth.
"

प्रकृतिं पुरुषं चैव विद्ध्यनादी उभावपि |
विकारांश्च गुणांश्चैव विद्धि प्रकृतिसम्भवान् || 20 || CH 13

prakṛitiṁ puruṣhaṁ chaiva viddhy anādī ubhāv api
vikārānśh cha guṇānśh chaiva viddhi prakṛiti-sambhavān

prakṛitim—material nature; puruṣham—the individual souls; cha—and; eva—indeed; viddhi—know; anādī—beginningless; ubhau—both; api—and; vikārān—transformations (of the body); cha—also; guṇān—the three modes of nature; cha—and; eva—indeed; viddhi—know; prakṛiti—material energy; sambhavān—produced by

Know that *prakṛiti* (material nature) and *puruṣh* (the individual souls) are both beginningless. Also know that all transformations of the body and the three modes of nature are produced by material energy.

The material nature is called Maya, or *prakṛiti*. Being an energy of God, it has existed ever since He has existed; in other words, it is eternal. The soul is also eternal, and here it is called *puruṣh* (the living entity), while God Himself is called *param puruṣh* (the Supreme Living Entity).

The soul is also an expansion of the energy of God. *śhaktitvenaivāṁśhatvaṁ vyañjayanti* (Paramātma Sandarbh 39.1)

"The soul is a fragment of the jīva śhakti (soul energy) of God." While material nature is an insentient energy, the jīva śhakti is a sentient energy. It is divine and untransmutable. It remains unchanged through different lifetimes, and the different stages of each lifetime. The six stages through which the body passes in one lifetime are: asti (existence in the womb), jāyate (birth), vardhate (growth), vipariṇamate (procreation), apakṣhīyate (diminution), vinaśhyati (death). These changes in the body are brought about by the material energy, called prakṛiti, or Maya. It creates the three modes of nature—sattva, rajas, and tamas—and their countless varieties of combinations.

Prakriti or Maya camouflages the reality. It is like a mirage often experienced by a traveller in the desert. Walking beneath a scorching Sun, dehydrated one does not find water anywhere. Suddenly in a distance, one sees an oasis of water and one rushes towards it only to discover that it was a mirage (मृगतृष्णा) and there is not even a drop of water. Adi Shankaracharya once remarked that the entire water in the oasis reflected by mirage cannot wet even one grain of sand.

Further, when the same traveller after walking a few steps looks back at the spot where he saw water earlier, he will still see an oasis. But now on he is not confused. Now he knows the truth and has experienced reality. He is enlightened. Gyan Yoga is quintessentially experiential, and Advaita Vedanta takes us through that experience to experience the truth for ourselves.

The fundamentals of Gyan Yoga are structured to investigate into our true self. It is kind of Self-inquiry and that by its very nature requires us to look inwards.

"Who looks outside dreams, who looks inside awakes".

It is an awakening that leads to enlightenment and life becomes an experience of pure bliss and reveals our identity which is "SAT-CHITTA-ANANDA.

There are four Mahavakyas, or great statements in the Upanishads, which have a profound significance as pointers to Reality. They are: (1) Prajnanam Brahma – Consciousness is Brahman; (2) Aham Brahmasmi – I am Brahman: (3) Tat Tvam Asi – That Thou Art; (4) Ayam Atma Brahma – This Self is Brahman.

The paradigm of Gyan Yoga essentially is concerned with us, the origin of the world, our relationship with the world, our true self, why are we here, what must we do, how should we act and purpose of life. Profound two worlds spoken by Christ "Know Thyself", become relevant.

It must be said that Vedanta answers these questions with great depth and understanding. While Vedanta espouses ancient knowledge which is of eternal significance, it must be enumerated in the context of the modern thought, and in the language that everyone can relate to. Otherwise, there is a danger of it becoming esoteric and somewhat abstract.

Vedanta unequivocally equates Self with Brahman. Everything in this universe is Brahman. Everything is the creation of Brahman; everything is the projection of Brahman and indeed, everything is Brahman. In other words, there is nothing in this universe except Brahman. Brahman is also described as universal consciousness which is only ONE that pervades the entire universe-every entity. This is most ancient wisdom and statement universally known as Advaita-Nonduality(अद्वैतवाद). While Brahman is only one, his creations and projections are many which is another name of Prakriti. All creations of Prakriti appear as Maya (माया).

ब्रह्मार्पणं ब्रह्म हविर्ब्रह्माग्नौ ब्रह्मणा हुतम् |
ब्रह्मैव तेन गन्तव्यं ब्रह्मकर्मसमाधिना || 24 ||

brahmārpaṇaṁ brahma havir brahmāgnau brahmaṇā hutam
brahmaiva tena gantavyaṁ brahma-karma-samādhinā

brahma—Brahman; arpaṇam—the ladle and other offerings; brahma—Brahman; haviḥ—the oblation; brahma—Brahman; agnau—in the sacrificial fire; brahmaṇā—by that person; hutam—offered; brahma—Brahman; eva—certainly; tena—by that; gantavyam—to be attained; brahma—Brahman; karma—offering; samādhinā—those completely absorbed in God-consciousness

Translation

For those who are completely absorbed in God-consciousness, the oblation is Brahman, the ladle with which it is offered is Brahman, the act of offering is Brahman, and the sacrificial fire is also Brahman. Such persons, who view everything as God, easily attain Him.

Commentary

Factually, the objects of the world are made from Maya, the material energy of God. Energy is both one with its energetic and different from it. For example, light is the energy of fire. It can be considered as different from the fire because it exists outside it. But it can also be reckoned as a part of the fire itself. Hence, when the rays of the sun enter the room through a window, people say, “The sun has come.” Here, they are bundling the sunrays with the sun. The energy is both distinct from the energetic and yet a part of it.

The soul too is the energy of God—it is a spiritual energy, called *jīva śhakti*. Krishna states this in verse 7.5.
Chaitanya Mahaprabhu stated:

jīva-tattva śhakti, kṛiṣhṇa-tattva śhaktimān
gītā-viṣhṇupurāṇādi tāhāte pramāṇa
(Chaitanya Charitāmṛit, Ādi Leela, 7.117) [v19]

“Lord Krishna is the energetic and the soul is his energy. This has been stated in *Bhagavad Gita*, Viṣhṇu Purāṇ, etc.” Thus, the soul is also simultaneously one with and different from God. Hence, those whose minds are fully absorbed in God-consciousness see the whole world in its unity with God as non-different from him. The Śhrīmad Bhāgavatam states:

sarva-bhūteṣhu yaḥ paśhyed bhagavad-bhāvam ātmanaḥ
bhūtāni bhagavatyātmanyeṣha bhāgavatottamaḥ
(11.2.45) [v20]

“One who sees God everywhere and in all beings is the highest spiritualist.” For such advanced spiritualists whose minds are completely absorbed in God-consciousness, the person making the sacrifice, the object of the sacrifice, the instruments of the sacrifice, the sacrificial fire, and the act of sacrifice, are all perceived as non-different from God.

The following two verses corroborate the statement above establishing the oneness of Brahman and everything else in the world is woven around Him and is just an appearance in consciousness.

मत्तः परतरं नान्यत्किञ्चिदस्ति धनञ्जय |
मयि सर्वमिदं प्रोतं सूत्रे मणिगणा इव || 7 || CH 7

mattaḥ parataraṁ nānyat kiñchid asti dhanañjaya
mayi sarvam idaṁ protaṁ sūtre maṇi-gaṇā iva

mattaḥ—than me; para-taram—superior; na—not; anyat kiñchit—anything else; asti—there is; dhanañjaya—Arjun, conqueror of wealth; mayi—in me; sarvam—all; idam—which we see; protam—is strung; sūtre—on a thread; maṇi-gaṇāḥ—beads; iva—like

There is nothing higher than Myself, O Arjun. Everything rests in Me, as beads strung on a thread.

Commentary

Here, Krishna states about His dominion and His Supreme position in this universe. He is the Substratum over which this entire creation exists; He is the Creator, Sustainer, and Annihilator. Like the beads strung in a thread, which can move in their place, God has given individual souls the free will to act as they wish, yet their existence is bound to Him. The Śhwetāśhvatar Upaniṣhad states:

na tatsamaśhchābhyadhikaśhcha dṛiśhyate
parāsya śhaktirvividhaiva śhrūyate (6.8)

"There is nothing equal to God, nor is there anything superior to Him."
In this verse, Krishna has clearly stated that He, in His original form, who stood before Arjun is the Ultimate Supreme Truth. By using the words, Me, My and I, He has dispelled the doubts that many have about Krishna Himself being God, the Supreme Lord, as many suppose that there is another higher formless entity, who is the ultimate source of even Krishna. As the first-born Brahma prays to Krishna:

īśhwaraḥ paramaḥ kṛiṣhṇaḥ sachchidānanda vigrahaḥ
anādirādir govindaḥ sarva kāraṇa kāraṇam (Brahma Samhitā 5.1)

"Shree Krishna is the Supreme Lord, who is eternal, omniscient, and infinite bliss. He is without beginning and end, the origin of all, and the cause of all causes."

अथवा बहुनैतेन किं ज्ञातेन तवार्जुन |
विष्टभ्याहमिदं कृत्स्नमेकांशेन स्थितो जगत् || 42 || CH 10

atha vā bahunaitena kiṁ jñātena tavārjuna
viṣhṭabhyāham idaṁ kṛitsnam ekānśhena sthito jagat

athavā—or; bahunā—detailed; etena—by this; kim—what; jñātena tava—can be known by you; arjuna—Arjun; viṣhṭabhya—pervade and support; aham—I; idam—this; kritsnam—entire; eka—by one; anśhena—fraction; sthitaḥ—am situated; jagat—creation

What need is there for all this detailed knowledge, O Arjun? Simply know that by one fraction of My being, I pervade and support this entire creation.

Commentary

Krishna's statement indicates that he has already answered the question. Now, of his own accord, he wants to tell something remarkable. Having revealed many amazing aspects of his splendour, he says that the magnitude of his glory cannot be judged even from the sum of what he has described, for the entire creation of unlimited universes is held within a fraction of his being.

Why does he make a reference to a fraction of his being here? The reason is that the entire material creation consisting of unlimited universes is only one-fourth of God's entire manifestation; the remaining three-fourths is the spiritual creation.

pādo 'sya viśhwā bhūtāni tripādasyāmṛitaṁ divi (Puruṣh Sūktam Mantra 3) [v32]

"This temporary world made from the material energy is but one part of the Supreme Divine Personality. The other three parts are his eternal abodes that are beyond the phenomenon of life and death."

Interestingly, Krishna is in front of Arjun, within the world, yet he reveals that the entire world is within a fraction of his being. This is like the story of Ganesh and Lord Shiv. Once, Sage Narada gave Lord Shiv a very special fruit. Lord Shiv's two children, Kartikeya and Ganesh both began demanding the fruit from him. Lord Shiv thought that if he would give it to any one of them, the other would think that their father was biased. So, Lord Shiv announced a competition for his two children. Whoever circumambulated the entire universe and came back to him first would get the fruit.

On hearing this, Kartikeya immediately started off to circumambulate the universe. He was athletically and powerfully built and decided to take advantage of it. In comparison, Ganesh had a plump body and felt he was handicapped in competing with his brother. So, Ganesh decided to make up for it by using his intellect. Lord Shiv and Parvati were standing there. Ganesh circumambulated them thrice, and then announced, "Father, I have done it. Please give me the fruit." Lord Shiv, "But how have you gone around the universe? You have been with us all the while." Ganesh said, "Father, you are God. The entire universe exists within you. If I have gone around you, I have gone around the entire universe." Lord Shiv had to agree that his son Ganesh was very smart, and indeed he had won the competition.

Just as Lord Shiv was standing in one place, and yet the entire world was contained in him, similarly, Krishna announces to Arjun that the entire creation, consisting of unlimited material universes, is held within a fraction of his being.

Samkhya Yoga recognizes the existence of Purusha and Prakriti. Advaita Vedanta recognizes the existence of only Brahman (Purusha). Both schools have their own very convincing stands, based upon observations, experience and strong logic. Gyan Yoga digs deep into the experience of every individual, and short of any direct evidence of the proof of existence of God (there can be none), it seeks to establish the identity of the Self as nothing but pure consciousness and everything that is visible, as appearance in that universal consciousness.

It would be worthwhile to examine deeply the tenets of Samkhya Yoga which at the face of it appears more real in our experience of the world as we perceive and indeed see. Purusha and Prakriti may verily be compared with the microcosm and macrocosm. Microcosm, representing the Purusha, individual consciousness, the Self, Soul or eventually Brahman. Macrocosm, the nature, the universe, galaxies, matter, energy, and all that we conventionally associate with nature with its bounty, full of beauty and wonder. The two phenomena may also be referred to as Subject and Object.

The sage Kapila, referred to as the first philosopher of humanity, who also propounded the essential principles of Samkhya Yoga, spoke about the Law of causality. According to this law, everything that happens in the world has a cause. All that we see is the effect of a cause. The creation of the universe, the big-bang theory and everything connected with creation, is preceded by a cause. Interestingly, the effect of the cause also becomes a cause for a subsequent effect. The entire universe this way, is bound by an unending chain of cause and effect. It is axiomatic to say that nothing comes out of nothing. We inexorably move from the unmanifest to the manifest. The famous example of chicken and egg story. While the debate is about which came first, we are concerned more about the chick being the cause of the egg and in time, egg becomes the cause of the chic and so on and so forth.

Another example relates to the link between the seed and the tree. Seed in earth sprouts into a tiny plant, and in time grows to become a tall tree with several branches, flowers, and fruits. The trunk of the tree provides support to the tree which can, depending upon the species, go up too many feet above the ground. Fruits on the tree ripen and in fullness of time break open and drop many seeds on the ground. The cycle begins all over again and this phenomenon goes on for several millennia. This process may be termed as evolution followed by involution and so forth. Interestingly, it never stops and does not require any external intervention.

What is more remarkable in this phenomenon is the diversity that is visible all around. There are millions of trees in every eco-system. There are similarities in some and huge variety in many others. Every seed carries a particular genetic code that will lead to the germination of that species and none other. This is true of all creation, right from human beings, animals, and plants, on ground and under water. There is no exception. Here the seed in an unmanifest state, manifests itself into a tree, an animal, a human, depending upon the genetic configuration intrinsic to its being.

Cause-effect-cause phenomenon results in unmanifest-manifest-unmanifest states.

Exactly in the same manner, as stated earlier, there exists a symbiotic relation between the Microcosm and the Macrocosm, Purusha and Prakriti, subject and object, subtle and gross.

Samkhya Yoga strongly professes the existence of Purusha and Prakriti as independent entities. Advaita (Non duality) Vedanta does not openly contradict this proposition but recognises the existence of only one entity-Purusha or Brahman. It emphatically seeks to establishes the oneness of the entire universe, with no second. Everything apart from Brahman, including all elements of Prakriti is only an appearance in Brahman, appearing as Maya. Gita in Chapter 6, verse 29 has this to say.

सर्वभूतस्थमात्मानं सर्वभूतानि चात्मनि |
ईक्षते योगयुक्तात्मा सर्वत्र समदर्शनः || 29 || CH 6

sarva-bhūta-stham ātmānaṁ sarva-bhūtāni chātmani
īkṣhate yoga-yuktātmā sarvatra sama-darśhanaḥ

sarva-bhūta-stham—situated in all living beings; ātmānam—Supreme Soul; sarva—all; bhūtāni—living beings; cha—and; ātmani—in God; īkṣhate—sees; yoga-yukta-ātmā—one united in consciousness with God; sarvatra—everywhere; sama-darśhanaḥ—equal vision

The true yogis, uniting their consciousness with God, see with equal eye, all living beings in God and God in all living beings.

Commentary

During the festival of Diwali in India, shops sell sugar candy moulded in various forms, as cars, airplanes, men, women, animals, balls, caps, etc. Children fight with their parents that they want a car, elephant, and so on. The parents smile at their innocence, knowing that they are all made from the same sugar ingredient, and are all equally sweet.

Similarly, the ingredient of everything that exists is God himself, in the form of his various energies.

eka deśhasthitasyāgnirjyotsnā vistāriṇī yathā
parasya brahmaṇaḥ śhaktistathedamakhilaṁ jagat (Nārad Pañcharātra)[v22]

"Just as the sun, while remaining in one place, spreads its light everywhere, similarly the Supreme Lord, by his various energies pervades and sustains everything that exists." The perfected yogis, in the light of realized knowledge, see everything in its connection with God.

Ashtavakra Gita, the purest text of Advaita Vedanta, echoes identical views on the subject. Verse 6 in Chapter says.

सर्वभूतेषु चात्मानं सर्वभूतानि चात्मनि ।
विज्ञाय निरहंकारो निर्ममस्त्वं सुखी भव ॥ 6 ॥

sarvabhūteṣu cātmānaṃ sarvabhūtāni cātmani |
vijñāya nirahaṃkāro nirmamastvaṃ sukhī bhava || 6 ||

Recognising oneself in all beings, and all beings in oneself, be happy, free from the sense of responsibility and free from preoccupation with "me".

मया ततमिदं सर्वं जगदव्यक्तमूर्तिना |
मत्स्थानि सर्वभूतानि न चाहं तेष्ववस्थित: || 4 || CH 9

mayā tatam idaṁ sarvaṁ jagad avyakta-mūrtinā
mat-sthāni sarva-bhūtāni na chāhaṁ teṣhvavasthitaḥ

maya—by Me; tatam—pervaded; idam—this; sarvam—entire; jagat—cosmic manifestation; avyakta-mūrtinā—the unmanifested form; mat-sthāni—in Me; sarva-bhūtāni—all living beings; na—not; cha—and; aham—I; teṣhu—in them; avasthitaḥ—dwell

This entire cosmic manifestation is pervaded by Me in My unmanifest form. All living beings' dwell in Me, but I do not dwell in them.

Commentary

The Vedic philosophy does not accept the concept of God creating the world and then peeping into it from the seventh heaven to check whether His world is running all right. They repeatedly propound the theme of God being all-pervading in the world:

eko devaḥ sarvabhūteṣhu gūḍhaḥ sarvavyāpī
(Śhwetāśhvatar Upaniṣhad 6.11)

"There is one God; He is seated in everyone's heart; He is also everywhere in the world."
īśhāvāsyam idam sarvaṁ yat kiñcha jagatyāṁ jagat (Īśhopaniṣhad 1)

"God is everywhere in the world."

puruṣha evedaṁ sarvaṁ, yad bhūtaṁ yachcha bhavyam (Puruṣh Sūktam)

"God pervades everything that has existed and all that will exist."

This concept of God being everywhere is understood subjectively. Some Eastern philosophers claim that the world is a *pariṇām* (transformation) of God. For example, milk is an unadulterated substance. In contact with acid, it transforms to yogurt. Thus, yogurt is a *pariṇām* (effect or product) of milk when it is transformed. Similarly, the protagonists of *pariṇām vāda* state that God has transformed into the world.

Other philosophers claim that the world is vivarta (to mistake one object for another). For example, in the darkness a rope may be mistaken for a snake. In the moonlight, a shining oyster may be mistaken for silver. Similarly, they say that there is only God and no world; what we are seeing as the world is Brahman.

However, according to verses 7.4 and 7.5, the world is neither pariṇām nor vivarta. It is created from the material energy of God, called Maya śhakti. The souls too are the energy of God, but they are His superior energy, called Jīva śhakti. Therefore, the world and all the souls in it are both God's energies and are within His personality. However, Krishna also says that He does not dwell in the living beings, i.e., the infinite is not contained by the finite beings. That is because He is far more than the sum of these two energies. Just as an ocean throws up many waves, and these waves are a part of the ocean, but the ocean is much more than the sum of the waves, similarly too, the souls and Maya exist within the personality of God, yet He is beyond them.

Gyan Yoga is essentially a journey to tell you who you really are. It introduces you to the methods of self-discovery, wherein you assume the role of a subject and everything outside you is an object. According to one definition, everything that objects to your consciousness is an object. Another way to look at this is that everything that you are aware of, is an object. The precepts of Gyan Yoga, an ancient science and wisdom, must be understood and explained in modern language, relatable to how we see and experience the world. It would be interesting to use three pointers to establish our identity.

Firstly, it is the **paradigm of Drashta and Drishya**, the seer and the seen. It is obvious, indeed logical to state that the seer and the seen cannot be the same. Eyes see an object, say a bottle. Clearly, eyes and the bottle are different. Also, eyes are seeing the bottle. Bottle is not seeing the eyes. Eyes are the subject, and the bottle is an object. It would be quite weird if the bottle were to say- hello eyes how are you? Another statement that the subject cannot be the subject for itself is equally logical. For example, eyes that are seeing the bottle which is placed away from it cannot see itself. We do and can see the eyes in a mirror, but that is only the reflection and not the eyes. Further, the experience of seeing the bottle is not in the eyes, which are only a glass formation through which light enters, and through the medium of the optic nerve, bottle is seen at the optic centre located in the brain.

In other words, our mind is aware of the eyes that are an instrument of seeing the bottle. We, our mind, and intellect are aware when eyes are open, when they blink and when these are shut. Applying the same logic, our mind becomes the subject and eyes an object. Eyes are not aware of the mind. Mind is aware of the eyes and through them, aware of the bottle. Our mind experiences all phenomena accorded to it by all five senses, namely, seeing, tasting, hearing, touch, and smell. Mind is the Drashta and all sensory experiences are Drishya. Apart from multiple sensory experiences, several other thoughts emanate in our mind in a constant unending stream, and in a manner that is incoherent and unconnected. Our mind being aware of the sensory experiences and thoughts, becomes the subject and the thoughts are objects. As a reaffirmation, mind is aware of the thoughts, thoughts are not aware of the mind.

There is another entity in our system which plays a stronger role in our existence, and possesses several higher attributes of memory, storage, and sense of discrimination. This is our intellect which guides our journey in performance of all our functions-thought, speech, and action, collectively described as our karmas. While our thoughts and several sensory experiences in the mind are induced by our connect with the external world, our intellect observes them and is aware of them. It is endowed with the faculty of independent thinking, a sense of right and wrong and helps us course through life with intelligence and wisdom. Intellect is aware of our mind and what goes on inside it and not the other way round. **Intellect is the subject, and the mind becomes an object.**

Beyond the intellect there is complete blankness or nothingness. All that has been described above and all that we are aware of, is verily illumined by our Consciousness. Vedanta summarises it as (Tat Tvam Asi) "Thou art that". All experiences of the body, senses, mind, and intellect are in our Consciousness. In other words, everything that is out there in the world is an appearance in our Consciousness. Our constant occupation bordering on our obsession with the outside world takes us away from reality. It is right there, but we fail to see it.

In spiritual circles, there is a popular story of the tenth man which is worth recounting.

Ten friends set out on a pilgrimage and had to cross a river on their journey ahead. They started and went across the other side. One of them suggested that we should take a count of all our friends to make sure everyone has crossed, and none is left behind. This person started the count from 1 to 9 and stopped after everyone was counted. Another person mentioned that there might be a mistake in counting and volunteered to count. He followed the same procedure and could not go beyond number 9. They started crying thinking that there are only 9 left and one of them is missing or has drowned. They sat there mourning the loss of one of their friends. Just then there was a wise man passing by and hearing them crying, asked the reason of their grief. They repeated the story saying that ten of them had set out for a journey and crossing the river one of them got drowned and only 9 are left. They are not sure whether they should continue their journey. Wise man meanwhile had done a quick mental count and saw that all ten were there and asked one of them to count again. Reluctantly, one of them got up and started counting one more time. He started from 1 and as soon as he reached number 9, he stopped. Everyone looked at the wise one askance. The passer-by held the hand of the one who was counting and turned it towards him and declared 'You are the tenth one". (Tat Tvam Asi), You are the tenth one and you are that. The parable demonstrates a very common occurrence and a fact that very often truth is right here in front of us, but we fail to see it.

Next pointer for establishing our identity or the real Self, relates to the changing-unchanging paradigm. Our body typically goes through seven stages of growth and decline. These are birth, growth, development, youth, maturity, decline and death. Body keeps changing every moment of its existence. Being a cellular entity, it keeps shedding old dead cells and keeps getting new ones, in accordance with the predetermined code, and through a biological process of cell division. The rate of cell division is faster in early years of growth and starts declining with age. According to one estimate, the total weight of the cells dropped by the body in one's lifetime is almost equivalent to 4.5 KG. We change more than one thousand skin bodies in our lifetime. We are given a name at the time of our birth and that stays with us till our death and beyond. Body changes constantly, our name and our identity does not change. Changes are happening in the physical body, in senses and the related experience, in our mind (Our thoughts keep changing all the time), our intellect becomes more mature, wiser with age (though not uniformly in all cases). The energy levels are perceptibly low, and all organs slow down. There comes a day in everyone's life without exception, when the last breath is taken, and the body becomes quiet. Our very existence (the gross form) is annihilated. The world continues to remember us by our name given to us at the time of birth.

While all these changes are happening incessantly, some perceptibly, some imperceptibly we remain aware of them all. Applying the same logic (The Seer and the seen) that if we are aware of something then it must be different from us. It is also important to note that the awareness of all the changes that are happening, or being experienced is on our side, and not on the side of body or mind where the changes are taking place. We are that witness-consciousness of the changes in us, in body, mind, intellect.

Thou Art That

The third pointer relates to the sentient and insentient element present in all living beings. The subtle and the gross (जड़-चेतन). A close appraisal of the elements present in our body will clearly establish the presence of two sets of entities-gross and subtle. To begin with, our body built with five elements such as, earth, water, fire, wind, and sky presents itself as a gross entity. It houses several organs such as nose, eyes, ears, tongue, and skin that give us sensory experiences. These symbols or organs are essentially gross entities but the experiences they bring is of a subtle nature and is not measurable. There are other organs in the body that are not outwardly visible but perform other necessary functions for living. Kidney, heart, pancreas, prostrate, liver and host of other minor and major organs that collectively collaborate to ensure healthy and active existence.

Sensory experience though facilitated by senses is experienced not at the sense level but at a corresponding centre somewhere in the brain, which connects with the sensory organ through a network of nerves. Nerves propelled by a mild electrostatic current, carries the message and gives us an experience of taste, smell, sight, touch, and sound. Here it is important to understand that it is always the sentient being that has awareness on its side, and not with the insentient being. In the current scenario, awareness lies with the mind or the intellect, which is the function of the brain and not with the sense organ, which is insentient and merely an instrument of communication. Here again, brain is an organ of the body and at best an instrument that facilitates the experience. Brain is gross and the intellect provides the subtle experience. Awareness is not on the side of the brain but is with the intellect. We move a step further and realise clearly that the experience of the intellect is known to another entity. We know our thoughts and have the capacity to change it. We as a person or a subtle entity don't change but it is possible for us to change the flow and the nature of our thoughts. We can take recourse to the changing-unchanging paradigm and the two must be different. Something other than the intellect is aware of that experience, or for that matter all experiences that pass through the domains of senses, mind, and intellect. We can apply the same logic of the seer and the seen. The experience of the intellect is experienced by us, and therefore it must be different from the intellect. That 'Us' or 'I' is defined by Vedanta as Tat Tvam Asi-You are that. That is pure consciousness and everything else that is being experienced, is only an appearance in our consciousness.

In the subject-object scenario, it is always better to start with experience which belongs to the subject. Experience is real, scientifically validated and is always on the side of the subject, never on the side of the object. An object is completely agnostic to who observes it and is amenable to different kinds of experiences for different people. We see a glass of water and the experience of seeing the glass is on our side and not on the side of the glass.

All experiences are illumined by our consciousness which remains unchanged while everything else including all our experiences are changing every moment.

Let us illustrate this with an example of a hall where many people are gathered. There are chairs, people sitting on them, a table, a glass of water on the table, a clock on the wall and many painting adorning the walls. There is a big bulb or a similar source of light on the ceiling that allows every object to be seen by everybody. Our eyes give us an experience of seeing people and objects in the hall. If someone speaks, our ears help us understand the words spoken. A handshake confirms the presence of another person through touch. Sitting inside the hall, even if some serious business is being transacted, different thoughts, not necessarily related to the subject arise and disappear. Our intellect absorbs the statements by speakers, internally forms a view and reacts to some of them.

Everything inside the hall is constantly undergoing changes, some visible that are gross, some invisible that are subtle-such as thoughts in our mind or those in others. The light above is illuming everything, every object in the hall but the light does not change. The light above also does not need another light to register its presence. It is self-illumined. That light is consciousness present in all of us. It is a witness of all that is present in the hall that is subject to change, but the light does not change. At an individual level that is also a witness of what is going inside our senses, mind, and intellect.

There is an interesting observation made by a doctor, a neurosurgeon. He said that during his profession, he treated several patients, looked deep into the brain, saw many MRI scans, but only thing that he could see were different parts of the body, organic stuff. He searched carefully for an entity called awareness, consciousness, or something like it, but could see nothing but the body, more body organic and gross. This is exactly what Vedanta says that you are somewhere in the body, part of it yet apart from it. You are different from your body. You are existence-consciousness-bliss, invisible but present everywhere. **Ashtavakra Gita** makes a direct statement in this regard.

न त्वं देहो न ते देहो भोक्ता कर्ता न वा भवान् ।
चिद्रूपोऽसि सदा साक्षी निरपेक्षः सुखं चर ॥ 4 ॥

na tvaṃ deho na te deho bhoktā kartā na vā bhavān |
cidrūpo'si sadā sākṣī nirapekṣaḥ sukhaṃ cara || 4 || CH 15

You are not the body, nor is the body yours, nor are you the doer of actions or the reaper of their consequences. You are eternally pure consciousness the witness, in need of nothing - so live happily.

The play of life goes on like a movie on the screen and we develop a tendency to start identifying ourselves with the film, its story, and the characters. All that is unreal but during the time we are sitting in a theatre, we are deluded in believing that it is real. We laugh, we cry, we sympathise, we empathise, we hate, we love, and our real thoughts are hijacked by the story that is being played on the screen. All that is happening in the movie is like the dream that we often see during our sleep. When we wake up or when we leave the theatre, we get back to the real world. Neither the dream nor the movie has any connect or any influence on our life. In a short while we forget both and the pressure and other important issues of life take over. We remain completely unaffected.

The character in the film is also playing his part dictated by the script and the director. If he is playing the role of a beggar or a billionaire, he does not become a beggar a billionaire in real life. If he is killed by the villain, he does not die. A child having just seen a film where the hero is killed, meets him in person and wonders what to believe.

There is an interesting story of a father and son going to see a film in a theatre. This was the first time for the son, though the father had seen many films before accompanying his son. It so happened that before the duo entered the cinema hall, the film had started. It was an action film with weapons, hills, rivers, and a few animals thrown in. Before leaving home, father had explained to the son some broad features of a movie where there is a screen in front, a projector that projects the film on the screen through powerful light and the viewer can have an experience that appears real. The film is based on a story, real or imaginary but characters are not real. They are only acting their part given to them by the director who decides on who will do or say what.

Son watched the film and the action in the movie made him sit on the edge and he seemed fully captivated by the events moving at a frenetic pace. Just then he remembered that his father had told him that there was a screen on which everything is projected and only then the viewers are able to see the film. He asked the father where the screen was and father replied-right there in front of you. Son evidently could not see the screen and repeated his question. Father gave the same reply. Son could only see the characters, objects, weapons and different locations, rivers, mountains et al. He pointed out to all of them and asked are those the screen. Father said, No right behind all of them. Son was not convinced and after a few more queries went back to watch the movie.

Suddenly, the movie stopped and in big bold letters, they could see the word "INTERMISSION". The lights came on dimly, but these were enough to see everything. Father quickly told the son- see there is the screen. Oh! that is the screen he yelled with excitement. The son now knew the screen and was happy and satisfied. After a while, the lights were dimmed and movie began, and the action started. This time the son watched the film completely absorbed and asked no questions. The screen became invisible again and one could only see the action, the story and all the characters that had gone away briefly during the interregnum. Once the movie was over, father and son came back happy. Soon everything was forgotten, and life came back to its normal track.

It was just a film but all that transpired inside the hall had some important takeaways. What was projected on the screen was like a dream that we sometime see during our dream sleep. It does not happen when we are awake, when everything that we see seems real. The screen only facilitates the movie to run and allows us to have the experience of seeing the film. Without the screen it would not be possible to see the film. This is exactly what happens in real life. We need a screen to experience all that is happening in our life and that screen is our consciousness. It is right there all the time for us to have experiences of different kinds that we go through every moment of our existence. Screen or our consciousness illumines everything, every object we see, every thought that rises in our mind, every person we meet. In short everything that occurs and indeed, all our experiences in our awakened or dream state are lit by our consciousness.

The screen is completely agnostic to what is being shown in the film. The same screen will show an action film, a horror movie, a romantic comedy and is completely unaffected by what is being shown. A river shown in the film does not wet the screen, fire in the building does not burn it, sword fight does not tear the fabric on the screen.

The screen is totally unaffected by what is going on in the film as being projected on it. This is also true of our consciousness which only lights up different experiences of our life without being affected by it one bit. The play of life as the movie, is going on at its own pace but our consciousness or awareness remains neutral to all our experiences. It plays the role of a facilitator without being involved or attached to anything. It is like a bulb in the ceiling that lights up all objects and people in the room. People and the objects in the room may change, shift, or move out but the bulb stays and shines unchanged.

It is interesting to notice in the story above that the screen (Consciousness) is invisible while the movie or the play of life is being played. The viewer is too deeply involved in watching the film to realise that all what is happening is merely an appearance on the screen. In between during the interval, screen appears and there is a flash of realisation. However, when the movie resumes, we are back into the state of ignorance of the existence of screen. Continual play of life keeps us in a state of relative delusion and ignorance.

All our life's experiences (these change constantly) are appearance in our consciousness which stays unchanged, unaffected, and pure.

यथा सर्वगतं सौक्ष्म्यादाकाशं नोपलिप्यते |
सर्वत्रावस्थितो देहे तथात्मा नोपलिप्यते || 33 || CH 13

yathā sarva-gataṁ saukṣhmyād ākāśhaṁ nopalipyate
sarvatrāvasthito dehe tathātmā nopalipyate

yathā—as; sarva-gatam—all-pervading; saukṣhmyāt—due to subtlety; ākāśham—the space; na—not; upalipyate—is contaminated; sarvatra—everywhere; avasthitaḥ—situated; dehe—the body; tathā—similarly; ātmā—the soul; na—not; upalipyate—is contaminated

Space holds everything within it, but being subtle, does not get contaminated by what it holds. Similarly, though its consciousness pervades the body, the soul is not affected by the attributes of the body.

The soul experiences sleep, waking, tiredness, refreshment, etc., due to the ego that makes it identify with the body. One may ask why changes in the body in which it resides do not taint the soul. Krishna explains it with the example of space. It holds everything, yet remains unaffected, because it is subtler than the gross objects it holds. Similarly, the soul is a subtler energy. It retains Its divinity even while it identifies with the material body.

यथा प्रकाशयत्येक: कृत्स्नं लोकमिमं रवि: |
क्षेत्रं क्षेत्री तथा कृत्स्नं प्रकाशयति भारत || 34 || CH 13

yathā prakāśhayaty ekaḥ kṛitsnaṁ lokam imaṁ raviḥ
kṣhetraṁ kṣhetrī tathā kṛitsnaṁ prakāśhayati bhārata

yathā—as; prakāśhayati—illumines; ekaḥ—one; kṛitsnam—entire; lokam—solar system; imam—this; raviḥ—sun; kṣhetram—the body; kṣhetrī—the soul; tathā—so; kṛitsnam—entire; prakāśhayati—illumine; bhārata—Arjun, the son of Bharat

Just as one sun illumines the entire solar system, so does the individual soul illumine the entire body (with consciousness).

Although the soul energizes the entire body in which it is present with consciousness, yet by itself, it is exceedingly small. eṣho 'ṇurātmā (Muṇḍakopaniṣhad 3.1.9) "The soul is very tiny in size." The Śhwetāśhvatar Upaniṣhad states:

bālāgraśhatabhāgasya śhatadhā kalpitasya cha
bhāgo jīvaḥ sa vijñeyaḥ sa chānantyāya kalpate (5.9)

"If we divide the tip of a hair into a hundred parts, and then divide each part into further hundred parts, we will get the size of the soul. These souls are innumerable in number." This is a manner of expressing the minuteness of the soul.

How can such an infinitesimal soul energize the body, which is huge in comparison? Krishna explains this with the analogy of the sun. Although situated in one place, the sun illumines the entire solar system with its light. Likewise, the Vedānt Darśhan states:

guṇādvā lokavat (2.3.25)

"The soul, although seated in the heart spreads its consciousness throughout the field of the body."

Synergies of the four paradigms

The four paradigms of Yoga discussed in different chapters in the book, address different states an individual finds himself in. Each of these forms if practised regularly with complete concentration and dedication, have the potential to live a life of fulfilment and achieve one's goal in life. At another level, all these forms are seamlessly connected with one another. Immersion in one form will inevitably lead to another. The process that needs to be followed would vary, but result is the realisation of truth, overcoming suffering and pursuing the path each one would choose for oneself.

One special and distinct characteristic of Gyan Yoga is that it must lead to realisation. Unlike others forms of yoga, you don't have to do anything. You must observe and experience the reality that lies intrinsically within you, something we fail to observe. There is an interesting story of a monk in the Himalayas, who spent several years studying scriptures, meditated day, and night, led a life of extreme austerity but somehow continued to feel inadequate, restless and was not sure whether he got anywhere close to realise the truth. He went to seek guidance of a senior monk who everyone said was already enlightened. The young monk described his story and all that he had been doing for several years but felt he had not achieved anything substantial in the spiritual domain. He asked what should he do now? The senior monk smiled and said yes what should you do now. It is not about doing anything; it is about realisation. In the sphere of knowledge, you are not required to do anything-you just need to realise by being a witness of the reality that you already are. (अहम ब्रह्मास्मि)

There is another story of a few junior renunciates who were recently admitted to the religious order and were give a mantra by their senior swami. They were required to chant that mantra several times. They did that for many years and one day decided to ask the senior monk as to how many times they should chant it in a day. The senior monk replied in a very sombre tone in a few words- "this mantra is not for chanting, it is for realisation, you may go now".

Bhakti Yoga needs preparation, fixing a daily routine, worshipping, be completely in love with your (इष्टदेव). You need to do something.

Karam Yoga is performance of your duties and remaining intensely engaged in your work without worrying over the rewards. You are doing something incessantly in an active mode, Dhyana Yoga or Raj Yoga requires great preparation before starting the process of meditation. The paradigm of Ashtanga Yoga has been extensively dealt with. You must do a lot, prepare yourself before you begin to get full benefits.

All these paradigms have one thing in common and that is complete purging of all impurities caused by reckless pursuit of material desires, purification of mind and intellect, and absolute surrender to Brahman. Indeed, Advaita Vedanta says that you already are that. You must know it, stay with it and accept it.

You then become the realised one. स्थितप्रज्ञ

Self-realisation does not happen on its own and it requires certain practices, discipline of the mind and self-control against numerous temptations created by Maya.

In chapter 13 of the Gita, Krishna spells out a very comprehensive regimen of practices that must precede the journey of self-realisation.

अमानित्वमदम्भित्वमहिंसा क्षान्तिरार्जवम् |
आचार्योपासनं शौचं स्थैर्यमात्मविनिग्रहः || 8 || CH 13

इन्द्रियार्थेषु वैराग्यमनहङ्कार एव च |
जन्ममृत्युजराव्याधिदुःखदोषानुदर्शनम् || 9 || CH 13

असक्तिरनभिष्वङ्गः पुत्रदारगृहादिषु |
नित्यं च समचित्तत्वमिष्टानिष्टोपपत्तिषु || 10 || CH 13

मयि चानन्ययोगेन भक्तिरव्यभिचारिणी |
विविक्तदेशसेवित्वमरतिर्जनसंसदि || 11 || CH 13

अध्यात्मज्ञाननित्यत्वं तत्वज्ञानार्थदर्शनम् |
एतज्ज्ञानमिति प्रोक्तमज्ञानं यदतोऽन्यथा || 12 || CH 13

amānitvam adambhitvam ahinsā kṣhāntir ārjavam
āchāryopāsanaṁ śhauchaṁ sthairyam ātma-vinigrahaḥ
indriyārtheṣhu vairāgyam anahankāra eva cha
janma-mṛityu-jarā-vyādhi-duḥkha-doṣhānudarśhanam
asaktir anabhiṣhvaṅgaḥ putra-dāra-gṛihādiṣhu
nityaṁ cha sama-chittatvam iṣhṭāniṣhṭopapattiṣhu
mayi chānanya-yogena bhaktir avyabhichāriṇī
vivikta-deśha-sevitvam aratir jana-sansadi
adhyātma-jñāna-nityatvaṁ tattva-jñānārtha-darśhanam
etaj jñānam iti proktam ajñānaṁ yad ato 'nyathā

amānitvam—humbleness; adambhitvam—freedom from hypocrisy; ahinsā—non-violence; kṣhāntiḥ—forgiveness; ārjavam—simplicity; āchārya-upāsanam—service of the Guru; śhaucham—cleanliness of body and mind; sthairyam—steadfastness; ātma-vinigrahaḥ—self-control;

indriya-artheṣhu—toward objects of the senses; vairāgyam—dispassion; anahankāraḥ—absence of egotism; eva cha—and also; janma—of birth; mṛityu—death; jarā—old age; vyādhi—disease; duḥkha—evils; doṣha—faults; anudarśhanam—perception; asaktiḥ—non-attachment; anabhiṣhvaṅgaḥ—absence of craving; putra—children; dāra—spouse; griha-ādiṣhu—home, etc; nityam—constant; cha—and; sama-chittatvam—even-mindedness; iṣhṭa—the desirable; aniṣhṭa—undesirable; upapattiṣhu—having obtained; mayi—toward Me; cha—also; ananya-yogena—exclusively united; bhaktiḥ—devotion; avyabhichāriṇī—constant; vivikta—solitary; deśha—places; sevitvam—inclination for; aratiḥ—aversion; jana-sansadi—for mundane society; adhyātma—spiritual; jñāna—knowledge; nityatvam—constancy; tattva-jñāna—knowledge of spiritual principles; artha—for; darśhanam—philosophy; etat—all this; jñānam—knowledge; iti—thus; proktam—declared; ajñānam—ignorance; yat—what; ataḥ—to this; anyathā—contrary

Translation

Humbleness; freedom from hypocrisy; non-violence; forgiveness; simplicity; service of the Guru; cleanliness of body and mind; steadfastness; and self-control; dispassion toward the objects of the senses; absence of egotism; keeping in mind the evils of birth, disease, old age, and death; non-attachment; absence of clinging to spouse, children, home, and so on; even-mindedness amidst desired and undesired events in life; constant and exclusive devotion toward Me; an inclination for solitary places and an aversion for mundane society; constancy in spiritual knowledge; and philosophical pursuit of the Absolute Truth—all these I declare to be knowledge, and what is contrary to it, I call ignorance.

Commentary

To gain knowledge of the *kṣhetra* and *kṣhetrajña* is not merely an intellectual exercise. Unlike bookish knowledge that can be cultivated without a change in one's character, the spiritual knowledge that Krishna is talking about requires purification of the heart. (Here, heart does not refer to the physical organ. The inner apparatus of mind and intellect is also sometimes referred to as the heart.) These five verses describe the virtues, habits, behaviours, and attitudes that purify one's life and illuminate it with the light of knowledge.

Humbleness. When we become proud of the attributes of our individual field, such as beauty, intellect, talent, strength, etc. we forget that God has given all these attributes to us. Pride thus results in distancing our consciousness from God. It is a big obstacle on the path of self-realization since it contaminates the entire field by affecting the qualities of the mind and intellect.

Freedom from hypocrisy. The hypocrite develops an artificial external personality. A person is defective from inside but creates a facade of virtuosity on the outside. Unfortunately, the external display of virtues is skin-deep and hollow.

Non-violence. The cultivation of knowledge requires respect for all living beings. This requires the practice of non-violence. Hence the scriptures state: *ātmanaḥ pratikūlāni pareśhāṁ na samācharet* "If you dislike a certain behavior from others, do not behave with them in that manner yourself."

Forgiveness. It is freedom from ill will even toward those who have harmed one. Harbouring ill will harms oneself more than the other. By practicing forgiveness, a person of discrimination releases the negativities in the mind and purifies it.

Simplicity. It is straightforwardness in thought, speech, and action. Straightforwardness in thought includes absence of deceit, envy, crookedness, etc. Straightforwardness in speech includes absence of taunt, censure, gossip, ornamentation, etc. Straightforwardness in action includes plainness in living, forthrightness in behaviour, etc.

Service of the Guru. Spiritual knowledge is received from the Guru. This imparting of divine knowledge requires the disciple to have an attitude of dedication and devotion toward the Guru. By serving the Guru, the disciple develops humbleness and commitment that enables the Guru to impart knowledge. Thus, Shree Krishna explained to Arjun in verse 4.34: "Learn the truth by approaching a spiritual master. Inquire from him with reverence and render service unto him. Such an enlightened saint can impart knowledge unto you because he has seen the truth."

Cleanliness of body and mind. Purity should be both internal and external. The Shandilya Upanishad states: *śhauchaṁ nāma dwividhaṁ-bāhyamāntaraṁ cheti* (1.1) "There are two types of cleanliness—internal and external." External cleanliness is helpful in maintaining good health, developing discipline, and uncluttering the mind. But mental cleanliness is even more important, and it is achieved by focusing the mind on the all-pure God.

māyādhīn malīn mana, hai anādi kālīn,
hari virahānala dhoya jala, karu nirmala bani dīn.
(Bhakti Śhatak verse 79)

"The material mind is dirty since endless lifetimes. Purify it in the fire of longing for God, while practicing utmost humility."

Steadfastness. Self-knowledge and God-realization are not goals that are attainable in a day. Steadfastness is the persistence to remain on the path until the goal is reached. The scriptures state: *charaivaite charaivate, charan vai madhu vindati* "Keep moving forward. Keep moving forward. Those who do not give up will get the honey at the end."

Self-control. It is the restraint of the mind and the senses from running after mundane pleasures that dirty the mind and intellect. Self-control prevents the dissipation of the personality through indulgence.

Dispassion toward the objects of the senses. It is a stage higher than the self-control mentioned above, in which we restrain ourselves by force. Dispassion means a lack of taste for sense pleasures that are obstacles on the path of God-realization.

Absence of egotism. Egotism is the conscious awareness of "I," "me," and "mine." This is classified as nescience because it is at the bodily level, arising out of the identification of the self with the body. It is also called the *aham chetanā* (pride arising out of the sense of self). All mystics emphatically declare that to invite God into our hearts, we must get rid of the pride of the self.

jaba maiṅ thā taba hari nathīṅ, ab hari hai, maiṅ nāhīṅ
prem galī ati sankarī, yā meṅ dwe na samāhīṅ (Saint Kabir)

"When 'I' existed, God was not there; now God exists, and 'I' do not. The path of divine love is very narrow; it cannot accommodate both 'I' and God."

In the path of *jñāna-yog* and *aṣhṭāṅg-yog*, there are elaborate *sādhanās* for getting rid of the *aham chetanā*. But in the path of *bhakti-yog*, it gets eliminated very simply. We add *dās* (servant) in front of *aham* (the sense of self), making it *dāsoham* (I am the servant of God). Now the "I" no longer remains harmful, and self-consciousness is replaced by God-consciousness.

Keeping in mind the evils of birth, disease, old-age, and death. If the intellect is undecided about what is more important—material enhancement or spiritual wealth—then it becomes difficult to develop the strong will required for acquiring knowledge of the self. But when the intellect is convinced about the unattractiveness of the world, it becomes firm in its resolve. To get this firmness, we should constantly contemplate about the miseries that are an inseparable part of life in the material world. This is what set the Buddha on the spiritual path. He saw a sick person, and thought, "O there is sickness in the world. I will also have to fall sick one day." Then He saw an old person, and thought, "There is also old age. This means that I will also become old one day." After that, He saw a dead person, and realized, "This is also a part of existence. It means that I too will have to die one day." The Buddha's intellect was so perceptive that one exposure to these facts of life made Him renounce worldly existence. Since we do not have such decisive intellects, we must repeatedly contemplate on these facts to allow the unattractiveness of the world to sink in.

Non-attachment. It means dispassion toward the world. We have only one mind and if we wish to engage it in pursuing spiritual goals, we must detach it from material objects and persons. The *sādhak* replaces worldly attachment with love and attachment toward God.

Absence of clinging to spouse, children, home, and so on. These are areas where the mind easily becomes attached. In bodily thinking, one spontaneously identifies with the family and home as "mine." Thus, they linger upon the mind more often and attachment to them shackles the mind to material consciousness. Attachment causes expectations of the kind of behaviour we want from family members, and when these expectations are not met, it leads to mental anguish. Also inevitably, there is separation from the family, either temporarily, if they go to another place, or permanently, if they die. All these experiences and their apprehensions begin to weigh heavily upon the mind and drag it away from God. Hence, if we seek immortal bliss, we must practice prudence while interacting with the spouse, child, and home, to prevent the mind from becoming entangled. We must do our duty toward them, without attachment, as a nurse does her duty in the hospital, or as a teacher does her duty toward her students in the school.

Even-mindedness amidst desired and undesired events in life. Pleasurable and painful events come without invitation, just as the night and the day. That is life. To rise above these dualities, we must learn to enhance our spiritual strength through detachment toward the world. We must develop the ability to remain unperturbed by life's reversals and not get carried away with the euphoria of success.

Constant and exclusive devotion toward Me. Mere detachment means that the mind is not going in the negative direction. But life is more than merely preventing the undesirable. Life is about engaging in the desirable. The desirable goal of life is to consecrate it at the lotus feet of God. Therefore, Krishna has highlighted it here.

Inclination for solitary places. Unlike worldly people, devotees are not driven by the need for company to overcome feelings of loneliness. They naturally prefer solitude that enables them to engage their mind in communion with God. Hence, they are naturally inclined to choosing solitary places, where they can more deeply absorb themselves in devotional thoughts.

Aversion for mundane society. The sign of a materialistic mind is that it finds pleasure in talks about worldly people and worldly affairs. One who is cultivating divine consciousness develops a natural distaste for these activities, and thus avoids mundane society. At the same time, if it is necessary to participate in it for the sake of service to God, the devotee accepts it and develops the strength to remain mentally unaffected by it.

Constancy in spiritual knowledge. To theoretically know something is not enough. One may know that anger is a bad thing but may still give vent to it repeatedly. We must learn to practically implement spiritual knowledge in our lives. This does not happen by hearing profound truths just once. After hearing them, we must repeatedly contemplate upon them. Such mulling over the divine truths is the constancy in spiritual knowledge that Shree Krishna is talking about.

Philosophical pursuit of the Absolute Truth. Even animals engage in the bodily activities of eating, sleeping, mating, and defending. However, God has especially blessed the human form with the faculty of knowledge. This is not to enable us to engage in bodily activities in a hedonistic way, but for us to contemplate upon the questions: "Who am I? Why am I here? What is my goal in life? How was this world created? What is my connection with the Creator? How will I fulfil my purpose in life?" This philosophic pursuit of the truth sublimates our thinking above the animalistic level and brings us to hear and read about the divine science of God-realization.

All the virtues, habits, behaviours, and attitudes described above lead to the growth of wisdom and knowledge. The opposite of these is vanity, hypocrisy, violence, vengeance, duplicity, disrespect for the Guru, uncleanliness of body and mind, unsteadiness, lack of self-control, longing for sense objects, conceit, entanglement in spouse, children, home, etc. Such dispositions cripple the development self-knowledge. Thus, Krishna calls them ignorance and darkness.

While several practices enumerated above are essential to gain knowledge, what is noteworthy in these five verses is the final declaration by Krishna in verse number 12. He says that constancy in spiritual knowledge and philosophical pursuit of Absolute truth is KNOWLEDGE, and anything that is contrary to it is Ignorance.

Living in the world, we are constantly called upon to act, to perform, attend to multiple responsibilities thrown on us by virtue of our unique station in life. There is no escape from these, but in the process, we get tied down to them and find it extremely difficult to get out or disengage. We remain perpetually attached and indeed, bound to our relations, friends, fame, power, and all material possessions. In such situation liberation becomes impossible, leave alone realisation or enlightenment. Strong attachments in the material world, lead to ignorance. The fundamental premise of Gyan Yoga is that we are free, not bound to anything, ever the witness and indeed, are Brahman. Without an abiding spiritual base, we remain constantly under a delusion that we are bound. The power to liberate ourselves lies only within us, but we refuse to exercise it out of fear of loosing out.

There is an interesting story that will illustrate this reality.

A washerman owned a donkey, and he would use it for carrying loads of clothes from his home to the riverside every morning. He would tie the donkey to the tree with a rope, offload the dirty clothes, go down to the river, wash the clothes, dry them up and before dark leave for home. Freshly washed and dried clothes were loaded on the donkey and after untying him, he would leave. This was his daily routine and his livelihood depended on this.

Like all other days, he reloaded the bag of clothes on the donkey's back and reached the tree where the donkey would be parked for the day. To his utter consternation he discovered that he had forgotten to bring the rope to tie the donkey with. He could not go back to fetch the rope because of the long distance to his home. Unable to leave the donkey in an untied position, as he was wondered what to do, a passerby saw him and asked him why was he so crestfallen. Washerman told him his predicament and asked for help. The passerby was a man of great wisdom and advised the washerman to park the donkey at the same place next to the tree, and as usual go through the motion of tying the donkey with the imagined rope. Washerman must make sure that the donkey is watching him while he is pretending to tie him. Seeing no other option, he proceeded to do as advised. He went through the motion of tying the donkey, removed the load from its back and went down to the river as usual. Carrying the bag of washed clothes, he began his climb with a fear in his heart about the presence of the donkey at the usual place. To his relief, the donkey stood where it always did, not moving an inch. He placed the bag on donkey's back and signalled it to move. Again, to his horror the donkey would not move. The washerman was stuck, and it was beginning to get dark. No amount of hitting or cajoling the donkey helped, it refused to move. Washerman went running to the wise man whom he had met in the morning and told him about this new situation. This time his advice was again very simple. He told the washerman to go through a similar movement of untying the rope from the tree, while ensuring that the donkey is watching him.

The washerman did not hesitate even for a moment and did as was advised. To his great surprise and indeed, relief, donkey started moving as always without any fuss.

We are not very different from the donkey in the story. Even when we are free from any shackles, we persist in believing that we are bound. We are forever free but obdurately refuse to accept or believe that we are free. The common refrain sometimes is that we are aware of this but are unable to unbind ourselves. Deluded by this belief, or an error in fully realising our true self, we stay perpetually bound and attached. This is Sansar, this is Maya and hence the cause of all sufferings in our life.

Life throws several opportunities for us to realise our true self, but the dust of ignorance, desires, attachment to the materiality cloud our vision. We are right there but are unable to recognise ourselves. There is an interesting story by the name of "Princess of Kashi" that illustrates this beautifully.

In the outskirts of the city of Varanasi, lived a king, his queen, and a five-year-old son. The queen got to know that some people in their kingdom were planning to stage a play by the name of Princess of Kashi. He called the director of the play and told him that her son who was young and good looking, would be ideally suited for that role. The young prince was chosen for the role, dressed up as a princess with necessary make-up and performed the role of the Princess of Kashi. He did a good job and was duly applauded for his performance. Those days photographic camera was not used, but artists and painter were commissioned to draw portraits of important people, actors, kings, queens and the rich folks who could afford it. The young prince dressed as the Princess had his portrait drawn and it was brought to the palace. Years passed by the young prince reached adolescence, became a tall youth with all the trappings of a prince, playing sports like horse-riding, shooting, archery and all that princes normally do.

One day he decided to go down to the cellar in the palace to look at the trophies, artifacts, paintings and all the gifts that normally are presented to the king by their subjects or other visiting royalties. While he was looking and casually moving around, he saw a painting of a young princess dressed up in her finery, looking gorgeous and extremely attractive. He stood transfixed and kept looking at the painting for a long time. He noticed that the painting was drawn about fifteen years ago; the date was engraved at the bottom. He guessed that the princess in the picture must be the same age as him now. After a while he was summoned for his meals but seemed to have lost his appetite. He fell in love with the princess whom he saw in the painting and looked lost and forlorn. He would not confide in his mother the queen, or his father the king, but continued to look lost as all young lovers are wont to do. The king and the queen were worried, but he would not share anything with them. One day an old inmate of the palace who was very close to the family asked the prince what the problem was. On persistent questioning, the prince confided that he was in love and ever since he had seen her, he cannot sleep, has lost his appetite, and desperately wants to marry her. On being asked about the identity of the lady he was in love with, he mentioned that he has never met her, but has seen her picture lying in the cellar of the palace. Whoever she is, she is so beautiful that he has fallen in love with her, only by seeing her picture. He can only dream of her beauty in real life. Ever since, he has been constantly thinking about her. The gentleman asked the prince to come down to the cellar and show him the picture.

The young prince pointed to the picture of the princess drawn fifteen years back. This person immediately recognized it and asked the princess to sit down. He told him the entire story and informed the prince that the portrait belonged to none other than the prince himself and was drawn fifteen years back after the play was staged. This realisation was enough for the prince to get back to his normal state.

"You are that". तत तत्वमसि

Ignorance of self creates delusion, leads to errors and becomes a cause of deep suffering. The prince was the victim of these syndromes and once knowledge dawned, he was cured of all his problems.

The greatest advantage of Gyan Yoga is that it gives an insight into who you really are. You were always that, but you did not see it. Even if you had sporadic flashes of realisation, you did not accept it as reality. Worldly desires and the stronghold of Maya pulled you back. You must believe in the reality of yourself, stay with it and remain in the state of perpetual bliss. You are "Sat-Chitta-Anand". Existence-consciousness-bliss. This is what Adi Shankaracharya repeated in in his beautifully composed "Nirvan Shatkam".

<u>चिदानंद रूप शिवोहम शिवोहम</u>

मनो बुद्धि अहंकार चित्तानि नाहं
न च श्रोत्र जिव्हे न च घ्राण नेत्रे |
न च व्योम भूमि न तेजो न वायु:
चिदानंद रूपः शिवोहम शिवोहम ||*1*||

[मैं मन, बुद्धि, अहंकार और स्मृति नहीं हूँ, न मैं कान, जिह्वा, नाक और आँख हूँ। न मैं आकाश, भूमि, तेज और वायु ही हूँ, मैं चैतन्य रूप हूँ, आनंद हूँ, शिव हूँ, शिव हूँ...]

I am not mind, nor intellect, nor ego, nor the reflections of inner self (chitta).
I am not the five senses.
I am beyond that.
I am not the ether, nor the earth, nor the fire, nor the wind (the five elements).
I am indeed, That eternal knowing and bliss, the auspicious (Shivam), love and pure consciousness.

न च प्राण संज्ञो न वै पञ्चवायुः
न वा सप्तधातु :न वा पञ्चकोशः |
न वाक्पाणिपादौ न च उपस्थ पायु
चिदानंदरूप :शिवोहम शिवोहम ||*2*||

[न मैं मुख्य प्राण हूँ और न ही मैं पञ्च प्राणों (प्राण, उदान, अपान, व्यान, समान) में कोई हूँ, न मैं सप्त धातुओं (त्वचा, मांस, मेद, रक्त, पेशी, अस्थि, मज्जा) में कोई हूँ और न पञ्च कोशों (अन्नमय, मनोमय, प्राणमय, विज्ञानमय, आनंदमय) में से कोई, न मैं वाणी, हाथ, पैर हूँ और न मैं जननेंद्रिय या गुदा हूँ, मैं चैतन्य रूप हूँ, आनंद हूँ, शिव हूँ, शिव हूँ...]

Neither can I be termed as energy (prana), nor five types of breath (vayus), nor the seven material essences, nor the five coverings (pancha-kosha). Neither am I the five instruments of elimination, procreation, motion, grasping, or speaking.
I am indeed, that eternal knowing and bliss, the auspicious (Shivam), love and pure consciousness.

न मे द्वेषरागौ न मे लोभ मोहौ
मदों नैव मे नैव मात्सर्यभावः |
न धर्मो नचार्थो न कामो न मोक्षः
चिदानंदरूप :शिवोहम शिवोहम ||3||

[न मुझमें राग और द्वेष हैं, न ही लोभ और मोह, न ही मुझमें मद है न ही ईर्ष्या की भावना, न मुझमें धर्म, अर्थ, काम और मोक्ष ही हैं, मैं चैतन्य रूप हूँ, आनंद हूँ, शिव हूँ, शिव हूँ...]

I have no hatred or dislike, nor affiliation or liking, nor greed, nor delusion, nor pride or haughtiness, nor feelings of envy or jealousy.
I have no duty (dharma), nor any money, nor any desire (kama), nor even liberation. (moksha).
I am indeed, that eternal knowing and bliss, the auspicious (Shivam), love and pure consciousness.

न पुण्यं न पापं न सौख्यं न दुःखं
न मंत्रो न तीर्थं न वेदों न यज्ञः |
अहम् भोजनं नैव भोज्यम न भोक्ता
चिदानंद रूप :शिवोहम शिवोहम ||4||

[न मैं पुण्य हूँ, न पाप, न सुख और न दुःख, न मन्त्र, न तीर्थ, न वेद और न यज्ञ, मैं न भोजन हूँ, न खाया जाने वाला हूँ और न खाने वाला हूँ, मैं चैतन्य रूप हूँ, आनंद हूँ, शिव हूँ, शिव हूँ...]

I have neither merit (virtue), nor demerit (vice). I do not commit sins or good deeds,
nor have happiness or sorrow, pain, or pleasure.
I do not need mantras, holy places, scriptures (Vedas), rituals or sacrifices (yagnas).
I am none of the triad of the
observer or one who experiences, the process,of observing or experiencing,

or any object being observed or experienced.
I am indeed, that eternal knowing and bliss, the auspicious (Shivam), love and pure consciousness.

न मे मृत्युशंका न मे जातिभेद:
पिता नैव मे नैव माता न जन्म |
न बंधू :न मित्रं गुरु :नैव शिष्यं
चिदानंद रूप :शिवोहम शिवोहम ||*5*||

[न मुझे मृत्यु का भय है, न मुझमें जाति का कोई भेद है, न मेरा कोई पिता ही है, न कोई माता ही है, न मेरा जन्म हुआ है, न मेरा कोई भाई है, न कोई मित्र, न कोई गुरु ही है और न ही कोई शिष्य, मैं चैतन्य रूप हूँ, आनंद हूँ, शिव हूँ, शिव हूँ...]

I am not afraid of death.
I have no separation from my true self, no doubt about my existence, nor have I, discrimination based on birth.
I have no father or mother, nor did I have a birth.
I am not the relative, nor the friend, nor the guru, nor the disciple.
I am indeed, That eternal
knowing and bliss, the auspicious (Shivam), love and pure consciousness.

अहम् निर्विकल्पो निराकार रूपो
विभुव्याप्य सर्वत्र सर्वेन्द्रियाणाम |
सदा मे समत्वं न मुक्ति :न बंध:
चिदानंद रूप :शिवोहम शिवोहम ||*6*||

[मैं समस्त संदेहों से परे, बिना किसी आकार वाला, सर्वगत, सर्वव्यापक, सभी इन्द्रियों को व्याप्त करके स्थित हूँ, मैं सदैव समता में स्थित हूँ, न मुझमें मुक्ति है और न बंधन, मैं चैतन्य रूप हूँ, आनंद हूँ, शिव हूँ, शिव हूँ...]

I am all pervasive. I am without any attributes, and without any form. I have neither attachment to the world, nor to liberation (mukti).
I have no wishes for anything because I am everything, everywhere, every time, always in equilibrium.
I am indeed, that eternal knowing and bliss, the auspicious (Shivam), love and pure consciousness.

Gyan yoga is the panacea of all our sufferings and the problems we encounter during our journey of life.

CHAPTER SIX

YOGA AND ENVIRONMENT

Yoga in everyone's life.

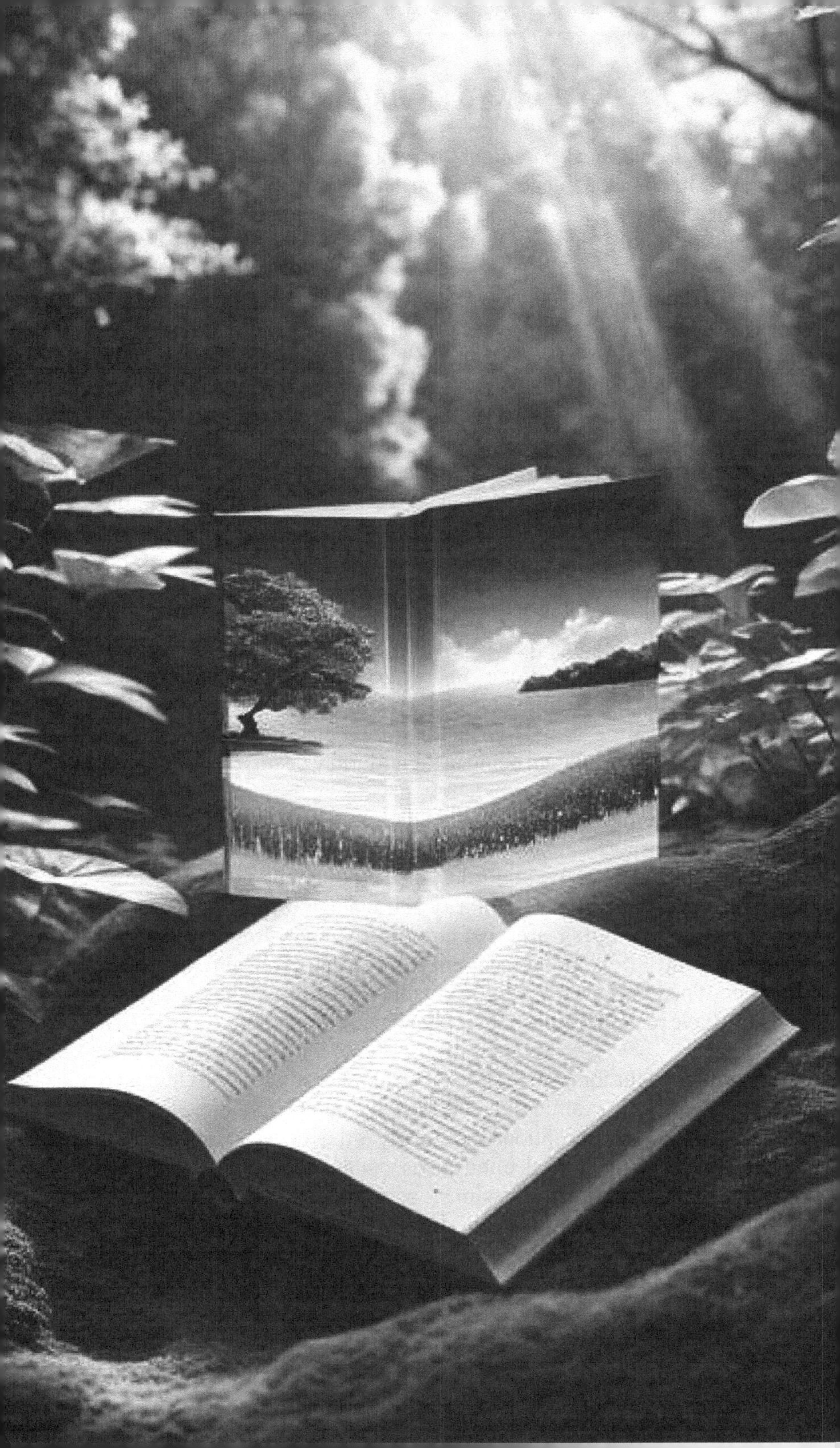

YOGA AND ENVIRONMENT

Practice of all classical paradigms of yoga are designed to create general wellbeing, happiness, freedom from suffering and equanimity at individual level. Yoga recognises every individual being as complete, a microcosm of Brahman and indeed, the most powerful means to realisation.

It is equally important to take a closer look at another dimension of Yoga, and that is its inclusivity and relevance for the entire mankind, nature, and the universe in its totality. This finds mention in the etymology of the word Yoga which literally translated means- "union", "joining". The next question that arises naturally is joining what. One needs two points or two entities for joining. Yoga again provides the answer which specifically refers to joining the internal with the external, or in yogic parlance-joining Purusha with prakriti. Here we need to take recourse to the tenets of Samkhya philosophy that recognises purusha and prakriti as separate entities. All experiences a human being goes through, is the result of a continuous interaction between the two.

Prakriti or external nature as we visualise it, has some very distinct notable attributes. These largely remain unchanged and are well-nigh predictable within a specified time frame. Five elements-Fire, earth, water, air, and sky are its principal constituents and five factors-time, space, matter, energy and free-will, impact every individual being in their journey on this planet.

In very simple terms, Yoga seeks to create complete harmony between Nature and all living beings-humans, animals, birds, insects, and all other cellular entities. Nature follows certain rules and seldom departs from them. We all need to respect nature for its seniority and vintage value. Some of its known and obvious attributes are, its continuity, ever-flowing, non-partisan behaviour, objectivity, ruthlessness in destruction, cyclical rejuvenation, and provider of needs of every living being on the planet. All these characteristics of nature have remained unchanged, ever since the creation.

The context is right for us to look at the general attributes of us human beings in contrast. A closer examination will reveal a completely opposite pattern of behaviour with a few exceptions. This really is the root cause of environmental degradation and ecological decline that is visible all over the world in terms of climate change, carbon emissions, ozone depletion and other related phenomenon that the world is experiencing lately. Human beings are driven not by a legitimate need but have been exploiting the resources of nature-earth, water, air, mineral resources, fossil oil under the influence of an uncontrolled greed. This process started with industrial revolution and has continued unabated with no signs of any reprieve for nature. Its impact is becoming visible in several parts of the world with increase in the mean temperature, melting of glaciers, dwindling of forest wealth. In brief, earth is in a state of danger, and unless strong corrective actions are taken to arrest the trend, entire mankind would be adversely affected. Increase in population and technological development, with more efficient means of exploitation has further aggravated the situation.

It is true that everyone is showing deep concern towards this development and international organisations, national governments are gearing up to take some measures to deal with the problem that is threatening to endanger the entire eco-system. It is important to realise that this problem has assumed such difficult dimensions that no effort is going to be adequate. Every citizen of this planet must work towards repairing the damage already done, as also perform acts for its restoration.

Here again, Yoga provides the answer. Its biggest mandate is to live in complete harmony with nature. Harness the resources of nature for sustenance and refrain from wilful destruction. Give back to nature that you take from it. Help in maintaining its pristine status for the benefit of the entire humanity, now and for posterity. Science of Yoga, at one level is essentially a form of practice by an individual and confers its benefits in building trust, love, selflessness, and knowledge. It also has strong community bonds in developing empathy for all living beings and helps in building an ethos where everyone treats others as equal. Every creation of nature is handled with respect ensuring long-term safety and sustainability of the environment.

Epilogue

Fundamentally, all paradigms of Yoga discussed above, lead to realisation, individually or collectively. They are indeed, seamlessly linked with one another. The practitioners are advised to choose any of them, immerse themselves into the chosen one fully, practise it and other forms would follow automatically. The path is not easy and demands perseverance, jettisoning worldly desires and seeking stability of thoughts and intellect.

Effort has been made, as is clearly visible from the text, to draw from the ancient knowledge encapsulated in scriptures such as Bhagwat Gita, Upanishads, Ashtavakra Samhita, Adi Shankaracharya's work and interaction with some known practitioners of various forms. Wherever possible a reference has been made for the readers to go to the original texts of these books, for further elucidation. With prayers on my lips and fervent hope in my heart, I sincerely believe that the readers will benefit from this work and in time, fully internalise the great wisdom of Yoga passed on to us by successive generations of great yogis.

This is indeed the most profound and valuable legacy given to us by our sages. It is upon us to practise it, spread it, share it with others and ensure that it keeps illuminating our minds in eternity.

Yoga is the most powerful guide in the evolutionary journey of mankind.

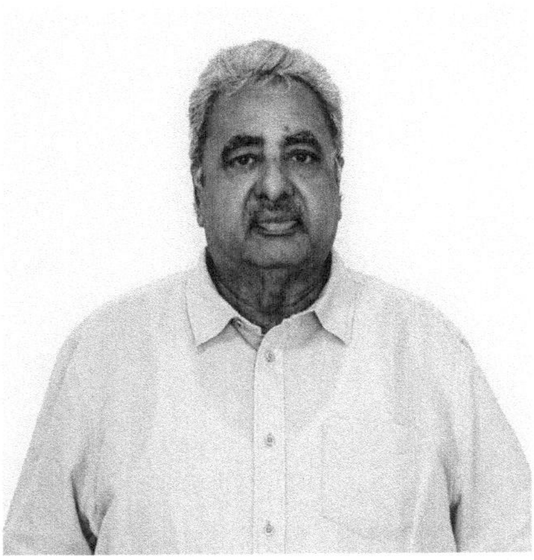

Having graduated in Physics from St. Stephen's College and with a degree of Law (Delhi University) and Management degree from UK, **Mr. Vinod Malhotra** joined the Indian Administrative Services. Had varied experience in diverse domains at the national and international levels. He also worked as an advisor to UNDP on certain projects relating to the field of art and craft. An avid reader and follower of Bhagwadgita, he envisioned a synthesis between Science and Spirituality.

He has written 25 books on different subjects covering Management, soft skills and leadership. His interest in music and fine arts led him to create musical compositions and poetry, largely in devotional genre. His lectures on spirituality, happiness, leadership and education are most sought after.

His deep and abiding interest in the science of Yoga led him to explore different paradigms of this ancient practice especially in the realms of lesser known areas like Bhakti, Karamyog and Gyan Yog.